SELF-CARE
FOR
Nurses

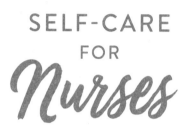

SELF-CARE FOR

Nurses

100+ WAYS TO REST, RESET, AND FEEL YOUR BEST

Xiomely Famighetti
BSN, RN, CCRN-CSC

ADAMS MEDIA
NEW YORK LONDON TORONTO SYDNEY NEW DELHI

▲**adams**media

Adams Media
An Imprint of Simon & Schuster, Inc.
100 Technology Center Drive
Stoughton, Massachusetts 02072

First Adams Media hardcover edition
November 2021

ADAMS MEDIA and colophon are
trademarks of Simon & Schuster.

For information about special
discounts for bulk purchases, please
contact Simon & Schuster Special
Sales at 1-866-506-1949 or
business@simonandschuster.com.

The Simon & Schuster Speakers
Bureau can bring authors to your
live event. For more information
or to book an event contact the
Simon & Schuster Speakers Bureau
at 1-866-248-3049 or visit our
website at www.simonspeakers.com.

Interior design by Julia Jacintho
Interior images © 123RF/Ekaterina
Bychkova

Manufactured in the
United States of America

1 2021

Library of Congress Cataloging-in-
Publication Data
Names: Famighetti, Xiomely, author.
Title: Self-care for nurses / Xiomely
Famighetti, BSN, RN, CCRN-CSC.
Description: First Adams Media
hardcover edition. | Stoughton, MA:
Adams Media, 2021.
Identifiers: LCCN 2021032183 |
ISBN 9781507217146 (hc) |
ISBN 9781507217153 (ebook)
Subjects: LCSH: Nurses--Job stress. |
Nursing--Psychological aspects. |
Stress management. |
Self-care, Health.
Classification: LCC RT86 .F36 2021 |
DDC 610.73--dc23
LC record available at
https://lccn.loc.gov/2021032183

ISBN 978-1-5072-1714-6
ISBN 978-1-5072-1715-3 (ebook)

Contents

CHAPTER FIVE: SOCIAL SELF-CARE..................................133

CHAPTER SIX: PRACTICAL SELF-CARE............................163

Introduction

Being a nurse can be rewarding, thrilling, and fulfilling—but it can also be *exhausting*. That's why you need to make time to take care of yourself just like you take care of your many patients.

So, why does it often feel difficult to muster up the energy and motivation to make this happen? Maybe you are busy with children or other family members to care for. Perhaps you feel guilt over prioritizing yourself, or you assume self-care would involve spending money you can't spare right now. Maybe you find it hard to switch gears from caring for others to caring for yourself.

As a nurse, you are asked to leave yourself at the door, put a smile on your face every day, and prepare to put your patients' needs first. You happily do this for hours at a time, and this is what makes it such a special profession. But you probably also tend to abandon your own self-care needs as you attentively focus on the well-being of patients and loved ones. It's time to start making *you* a priority.

That's where *Self-Care for Nurses* comes in! Throughout this book, you will learn how to sustain your physical, emotional, and mental health as a nurse, while also maintaining the practical aspects of daily life, keeping up with your social life, and developing a fulfilling professional career. You'll find over one hundred self-care activities to help you enjoy your life's meaningful work while also maintaining a balanced lifestyle once your shift is over.

Here are just some of the activities in this book:

- Use a gratitude journal to boost your mood and build a positive mindset.
- Exercise your mental muscles by learning something new, unrelated to nursing.
- Nourish your body by planning healthy work snacks in advance.
- Avoid professional burnout by learning how to say no to unwanted overtime.
- Revel in time with friends by hosting a game night.
- Do away with clutter that is causing you more stress.
- And more!

Prioritizing your own needs can be one of the keys to a successful and joyful nursing career. So, grab your favorite cup of brew, get cozy, and turn the page to experience rejuvenating self-care!

CHAPTER ONE

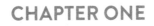
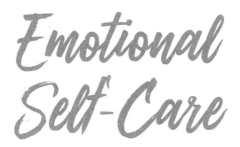

Emotional
Self-Care

We all have emotional needs that require nurturing. We need to be able to feel our feelings—both positive and challenging—and process them in a healthy way.

Nurses regularly open themselves up to be able to respond emotionally to their patients' issues, concerns, and struggles. Whether it's sharing the low of receiving a difficult diagnosis or the high of a treatment that worked as planned, emotional moments happen frequently during your days at work. But when you are constantly involved in other people's feelings, it can be challenging to switch gears and put your own emotions first sometimes. Prioritizing your emotional needs involves taking the time to feel positive emotions and learning how to deal with the negative ones. In this chapter you will learn how to make sure you're tending to your own emotional needs.

Some of the activities in this chapter will allow you to learn more about yourself and explore feelings you didn't know were lingering. These simple practices are meant to be repeated as often as needed and carried on long term in your nursing career and everyday life. A few emotional self-care ideas you will find in this chapter are sending yourself flowers, making a nostalgic meal, creating a playlist for various moods, creating a gratitude journal, and practicing self-forgiveness. Performing emotional self-care might feel unfamiliar at first, but it is a transformative experience that will leave you feeling happier and more fulfilled as a caretaker for others.

WRITE A LIST OF YOUR ACCOMPLISHMENTS

It's all too easy to let your busy day-to-day life consume you, making you forget all of the great things you have done in the past...and how much you have grown. Sometimes all you need is a quick reminder by writing them down in a list. This emotional self-care activity can help restore happiness, boost your confidence, and build a sense of pride in all you've accomplished.

The idea is as simple as it sounds: Write down a list of personal accomplishments you've made over the past five years. Some examples of things you might want to include on this list are passing a difficult exam, graduating nursing school, getting an award at work, staying healthy, learning a new skill, taking on new responsibilities, or even finding time for a weekend getaway with your family. No accomplishment is too small!

Once you've made your list, try to review and update it periodically. That might mean once a week or once every few months—whatever works for you.

The beauty of this activity is that it celebrates your wins and reminds you how amazing you are. This method of self-love can also motivate you to reach future goals. After all, if you achieved something difficult once, you can absolutely do it again!

CREATE A
GRATITUDE JOURNAL

Nurses have so much to be thankful for, but you might not always recognize it. Learning how to cultivate more gratitude in your life is a very powerful way of creating a happier, healthier, and more emotionally balanced you! Practicing gratitude is about reflecting on things you deeply appreciate, big or small.

As a nurse, you might find yourself focusing on negative outcomes since you see them regularly during your work hours. The constant scanning of your environment, looking for the next obstacle or problem, can quickly have you defaulting to negative thinking and a focus on what's lacking. Writing in a gratitude journal will help you turn your attention to the positives, the upside, and the solutions.

Writing in a gratitude journal can be as simple or as complex as you want to make it. Here's how to do it:

1. **Decide where and how you want to write.** You might choose a simple notebook or a decorative journal, an app on your phone, or your laptop.

2. **Choose a time that works best for you.** Whatever time feels right to you is the best time, whether it's first thing in the morning, once a week, after a shift, or whenever you choose.
3. **Get writing.** Set aside ten to twenty minutes to document one thing you are grateful for, followed by five reasons why. Some obvious areas to focus on are your family, health, friends, career, or home. But try being more specific, like feeling grateful for the specific way your pet greets you after a long day at work.

Your gratitude journal can help you find perspective and develop a deep sense of what it is like to be thankful for even the smallest things around you. Challenge yourself to be grateful even on your most difficult days. Creating a habit of acknowledging your gratitude will encourage you to recognize and appreciate all your many blessings as you deal with the emotional ups and downs of nursing.

LISTEN TO AN
AUDIOBOOK BEFORE BED

Nurses depend on good-quality sleep to perform optimally at work. You must walk in with sharp focus, quick memory recall, and a lot of physical energy. You have no time to feel tired and drained, right?

Unfortunately, like many other people, you might have trouble falling asleep sometimes, even though you're exhausted. Whether you're thinking about the shift you just had or your to-do list for tomorrow, a busy mind can hinder sleep. Both your emotional and physical health can suffer tremendously with lack of sleep, which will only make everyday stressors seem that much more difficult.

One of the most effective tools for getting a good night's sleep is to develop a calming nighttime routine. Reading is an excellent way to relax, but if you find yourself too tired to even hold a book open, try listening to an audiobook instead. You can choose short stories or meditations from mobile apps like Calm and Headspace that are easily accessible and meant to lull you to sleep. Or opt to listen to an audiobook from your favorite author. Look for a book that is not scary or too thrilling and is narrated by a tranquil voice. This will help you focus on the narrator and allow your own thoughts to fade away.

Drifting off to dreamland with the help of a recorded story may be the ticket to waking up feeling fresh and emotionally restored the next morning.

WATCH A COMEDY SPECIAL

They say laughter is the best medicine, right? We've all experienced how laughing and humor are beneficial for your emotional and mental health. Laughter can alter the neurotransmitters in the brain, dopamine and serotonin, consequently improving your mood. Plus, laughing can boost immunity, lower stress hormones, decrease pain, relax your muscles, ease anxiety and tension, and aid in preventing cardiovascular disease. Talk about an amazing emotional self-care technique!

Have you ever finished watching a funny video or meme with a colleague on your lunch break, and then suddenly realize that you can't remember what you were stressing over a few minutes ago? Nurses often use humor as a coping mechanism because it's a quick and easy way to improve your emotional well-being. Watching comedy specials regularly is a great way to keep humor in your day-to-day life.

Finding a comedian that matches your sense of humor is simply a matter of trial and error. You could start by watching short video clips online, then narrow it down to a few comedians that catch your interest. After you've chosen one that suits your style, check out one of their comedy specials, which can be up to ninety minutes long. If you don't have that much time, it's okay—just watch a few jokes and then pause and return to the special later. The bottom line is that incorporating laughter into your evening can help you return to joy if you've had a difficult day at work.

DO A FIVE-MINUTE MEDITATION BEFORE YOUR SHIFT

Heading into a long shift can feel daunting. Your emotions could range from excited to fearful to motivated. Your heart is palpitating and your mind is racing with anticipation. You are thinking of what events could possibly come to pass over the next several hours. You are not alone in this; all nurses experience pre-shift jitters.

Meditation is a powerful tool to help you manage stressful moments just like this. Meditating doesn't have to be done cross-legged on a peaceful mountain—you can try simple meditations like this one almost anytime, anywhere. Taking a few moments to center yourself and breathe slowly will help you prepare emotionally for anything your day has to offer. This five-minute meditation is quick and effective, and can be done in your car once you've arrived at work or on the train or bus as you head to work. So, let's get started.

- Safety comes first! If you have driven to work, put the car in park, lock your doors, and be aware of your surroundings. If you are taking public transportation, make sure your belongings are secure, your eyes are open, and you are able to hear what is happening around you.
- Get yourself in a comfortable position with both feet on the ground and your palms resting on your lap.

- Set an alarm for five minutes.
- Turn off any distracting entertainment like music or podcasts. That said, if there is too much noise around you, find soothing meditation or spa music (without lyrics) that you can listen to. You can use headphones if that feels comfortable to you.
- Close your eyes and inhale deeply.
- Feel the breath in your belly, and then feel it move up into your ribs, then your chest, and finally up to the crown of your head.
- Gently hold your breath for five seconds.
- Slowly reverse this process on the exhale for another count of five.
- As you breathe and hold, try to clear your mind. Rather than trying to "think of nothing," focus instead on being present in the moment and counting your breaths. If a negative thought comes to mind, acknowledge it and let it go, then return to the here and now.
- Continue this process for five minutes. When your alarm sounds, open your eyes. Enjoy your more relaxed and emotionally prepared mindset.

One of the most valuable benefits of practicing regular meditation is that it can build resilience over time—but it also has the capability of relieving anxiety in minutes, as shown in this activity. Try it before your next shift!

MAKE A NOSTALGIC MEAL

Nostalgia can provide comforting, reassuring emotions when you need them most. As a nurse, you might see the effects of nostalgia firsthand when a patient shares a special memory or story from their past. Their smile can easily turn into a giggle that develops into a full belly laugh. How amazing is that to witness?

You can evoke that same pleasant feeling by making a delicious recipe that reminds you of a happy memory. Whether it's a warm soup your grandparent made to warm you on cold days or a unique dessert your family served to celebrate special events, whipping up a dish that you associate with good times can help you recapture those happy memories. Since you're already probably overworked, you might not want to take on anything *too* difficult—the simpler and faster, the better.

As you savor the dish, try to connect with each of your five senses. Let the flavors, aromas, and textures take you back to that happy time and infuse you with those joyful emotions you shared with people you love.

SEND YOURSELF FLOWERS

Don't you love the feeling of walking into a patient's room and seeing fresh flowers at the bedside? Or coming home to a beautiful bouquet on your dining room table?

There's something special about fresh flowers' ability to lift your mood. Research has shown that keeping fresh flowers indoors may help with concentration and memory because the extra oxygen they provide fills up your living space and boosts your brain cells. Floral scents can also play a role in combatting the blues and lowering stress. Soothing scents like the ones from the flowers of lavender, chamomile, and jasmine are a few examples of calming aromatherapy.

You don't need to wait for a partner or loved one to send you flowers, though. Take the initiative and choose some yourself! You worked hard all week, keeping all of your patients safe, and now you want to remind yourself of how special and deserving you are.

You can hop online and get a bouquet delivered, visit a florist, or shop at your local grocery store and get creative building a bouquet of your own. The most important part of this activity is to do it with intention. Choose your favorite colors and soothing scents so the display is sure to brighten your spirits.

Don't forget to write yourself a lovely note to go along with it... from you to you, celebrating all of your hard work and dedication!

ACKNOWLEDGE
TRAUMATIC EXPERIENCES

Too often nurses work shifts that traumatize us emotionally, mentally, and physically. But how often do you go home and digest what actually happened?

It is easy as a nurse to fall into the habit of compartmentalizing while at work—but you may never actually process your feelings later. You constantly deal with stressors and trauma, but may brush it off as "this is just what I do." And in some senses, that's true—in order to effectively perform in any emergency situation, you need to master your parasympathetic nervous system and focus on what needs to be done in that moment.

After your shift, however, it's important to allow yourself to process your emotions in a healthy way. You are still human after all, and at the end of the day, what happens to you at work becomes a part of your life experience and will ultimately affect you as a whole.

Acknowledging your emotions may feel uncomfortable at first, but it's worth practicing. Here are two relatively easy ways to allow yourself to feel your feelings:

1. **Decompress before you arrive at home.** If you know your house is chaotic and will require lots of energy as soon as you walk in, take five minutes to sit in your driveway (or park down the street) to digest your day. Use this time to think about the events that took place during your shift, take note of the emotions that are coming up, and remind yourself that it is okay for you to feel this way. Take a few deep breaths and then make your way inside.

2. **Write down your feelings.** Once you are in a comfortable space after your shift, write down what actually happened and ask yourself: How am I feeling? Why do I feel this way? Could I have done anything differently to change the situation? After the questions are answered and you have acknowledged your shift, thank yourself for opening up and then feel free to let the emotions go and move on with your evening.

This activity helps you carve out space and time to face difficult feelings head-on so you can free yourself from them.

GET OUT IN NATURAL SUNLIGHT

When you're regularly working inside a hospital, office, school, or operating room for long hours, you can easily miss the chance to enjoy sunlight. You may even go into work before sunrise and leave work in the same darkness. Unfortunately, if you often miss out on sunlight, your emotional health is likely to suffer a bit.

Safe sun exposure has many mood-lifting and health benefits. For example, exposure to sunlight triggers production of serotonin in your brain, which is associated with mood-boosting and calming qualities. Safe amounts of sunlight also improve vitamin D production in your skin, which can ultimately build stronger bones, aid in preventing certain cancers, help heal some skin conditions, and improve immunity.

The good news is that you only need a few minutes here and there to grab some safe sun exposure. For example, you could take a ten- to fifteen-minute break outside in the sun, enjoy your lunch break outside, go for a quick walk with a coworker, or drink some of your morning coffee outside. You can also open up all the shades and blinds in your home and eat a picnic outside on your off days. Though you can't get vitamin D through the window, just being in the presence of the natural light can improve your mood.

Try to find those snippets of time during your workday to spend a few minutes basking in natural light. You will be surprised at how it can impact how you think, look, and feel!

COLOR IN A COLORING BOOK

That's right—coloring books aren't just for children anymore! There is no doubt that you live in a go, go, go state at work. Long shifts can leave you emotionally drained and without the energy to do much when you get home. Instead of plopping in front of a mindless TV show, consider coloring for a few minutes.

Coloring has many benefits that are important to nurses' emotional well-being. Coloring can help you slow down your thoughts and focus on the present moment—a practice known as mindfulness. Taking twenty minutes a week to color can induce a Zen-like state similar to what you'd accomplish with traditional meditation! Drawing and coloring also have the ability to relax the amygdala, the part of your brain that controls fear. Who knows fear and worrying better than nurses? After all, you are constantly anticipating the next diagnosis, intervention, admission, or task. Concentrating on coloring positive images can also help you get rid of negative thoughts.

No matter what your interests, you can find a coloring book that is perfect for you. Whether it's images of vintage flora, inspirational quotes with fun lettering, or geometric patterns, choose something that speaks to you. Grab some colored pencils, markers, or high-quality crayons, find a quiet spot, play relaxing music, and bring joy to your page. Let your inner child run free and start coloring without judgment!

CHALLENGE YOUR NEGATIVE THOUGHTS

Most people spend an enormous amount of time "inside their mind," especially nurses. Of course, a big chunk of your day involves thinking: thinking about your patient's diagnosis, what their medications are used for, how you will complete all of your tasks in a timely manner, and what family members you need to update. Even on your best and brightest days, your mind gets flooded with a mixture of your own commentaries.

Amidst this running narrative, negative thoughts can easily dominate. Maybe you're worrying about the future, replaying something that happened in your past, doubting yourself, or concerned about a patient or family member. While these worries might feel valid in the moment, too many negative thoughts can have a detrimental impact on your emotional health.

The key is to know which negative thoughts aren't worth your energy. The method of dealing with negative thoughts described here will help you learn to notice your negative thoughts, analyze whether they are actually as bad as you think, and replace them with truthful ones. Essentially, you are going to take five or ten minutes to challenge the legitimacy of your negative thoughts.

Start by drawing three big boxes on a piece of paper labeled *My Negative Thought*, *My Evidence*, and *My Conclusion*. In the first box, write down the negative thought that has been disturbing you. In the second box, list all of the evidence you have in your life to prove that this thought is true and real. In the last box, come to your conclusion, using your evidence, to credit or discredit the negative thought. For example, a negative thought can be "I am never going to get into the Nurse Practitioner program at my preferred school." The evidence you have to make this statement true would have to be a rejection letter from the program. If you don't have this evidence, your conclusion would be that this statement is false and based on fear. Therefore, part of your conclusion will be to turn the negative statement to "I have worked hard to be the best candidate I can be; if I don't get in, it doesn't mean that I am a bad nurse or that I am not going to get in at a later time." Arriving at your conclusion requires you to find evidence that proves the negative thought true. Take some time to reflect on the evidence that refers specifically to the thought.

What you'll likely realize is that most of your negative thoughts are not based on facts, but instead originate from fear and imagination. This step-by-step process will ultimately help you reframe your mind so that recurrent negative thoughts that aren't true don't use up your precious emotional energy.

JOIN A SUPPORT GROUP

Nurses (and nursing students!) carry a lot on their plates. Juggling your professional, personal, and social lives can be difficult. Even if you are surrounded with love and encouragement from the people in your life, sometimes emotional support from a group of strangers can be incredibly helpful.

Therapy is not just for big life crises, mental health diagnoses, and couples. It can be beneficial for anyone! Support groups can be an easy way to try out therapy (if you're still unsure, ask a like-minded friend to join with you). These groups are intended to be a safe, judgment-free place to acknowledge what you're doing right, reflect on current struggles you're facing, and come up with solutions with an unbiased group of strangers. This is a time for you to work on yourself alongside a set of people who have similar goals as you. Look online for a support group in your area that's targeted to your specific needs. There are plenty of groups for nurses, nurses who are parents, nurses in oncology, hospice nurses who constantly deal with loss, and more. If your work is going well and your main struggles are in your personal life, there are groups for that too.

Working with a support group will allow you to preserve and boost your emotional health. Not only will you be able to share emotions and vent, you can also receive encouragement and motivation from other members—and give it back to them too!

CREATE PLAYLISTS
FOR VARIOUS MOODS

Music has the amazing power to evoke emotional responses. Whether you're feeling sad, stressed, happy, or just bored, you can find music that can either match or improve your mood. Maybe when it's time to conquer a tough workout at the gym your go-to is hip-hop, but on your commute to work you need slow country music for stress relief. The beauty of music is that it comes in various flavors for various moods.

Invest some time in personalizing a few different playlists that you can easily access when you need them. You can label each playlist depending on the mood they are intended for, such as pre-shift mood booster, post-shift chill vibes, morning stretch, mid-shift walk, or study mode. Apple Music and Spotify are a couple of music platforms that make it simple to build playlists. Have fun with this exercise—you'll be thanking yourself later when you have just the right songs for your mood.

DO SOMETHING FUN TO IMPROVE YOUR MOOD

Doing something fun can help you get your mind off work, boost your mood, and revive your soul. Nurses spend so much time worrying about the health of others, and not enough time on their own. Refill your emotional health cup by doing something that excites you! A fun activity will help boost your overall creativity, energy, and productivity, and improve your outlook on life.

Fun has a different meaning for everyone, so think about what brings you joy. Doing something fun doesn't require you to spend lots of money or time, either. There are so many activities to choose from—here are some ideas:

- Eat at a new restaurant with an unconventional spin, like having a live band or cooking the food in front of you.
- Plan a poker night.

- Turn on happy music and dance while you get ready for work.
- Go to an outdoor group fitness class with friends.
- Rent a paddleboard or kayak.
- Go to a concert or out dancing with friends.
- Stay in and take a virtual painting class.
- Plan a themed cultural night.
- Jump on a trampoline.
- Head to a batting cage or driving range for some practice.
- Have an ice cream sundae buffet for dessert.

No matter what you choose, enjoy the happy and relaxed feelings that this activity brings you. Try to encourage this pleasant emotional state to stay with you as long as possible.

PRACTICE SELF-FORGIVENESS

Nurses tend to be very hard on themselves. It becomes second nature to put others first, strive for perfection, and overanalyze your performance at work. The main goal for each shift is to keep patients safe and healthy while not making any errors; unfortunately, that isn't always the case. Even the best nurse makes a mistake once in a while—you're only human.

Let's say you made a medication error and immediately alerted the doctors, the charge nurse, and your manager. You took the corrective actions and your patient is now safe. There's an invaluable lesson to be learned: You have made a mistake and can perhaps take action to see that it doesn't happen in the future (maybe you need to triple-check the order or the bottle before administering the medicine). What's key to remember is that a mistake doesn't make you a bad nurse.

Once you've dealt with the logistics of the mistake, it's time to deal with the emotional ramifications. Chances are, you're being very hard on yourself, replaying the event over and over in your head, and telling yourself all sorts of terrible things. To break up this negative self-talk, you need to forgive yourself. Practicing self-forgiveness is an important part of the journey to connecting with your true self and working on your emotional health. Learning to let go of past mistakes both at work and in your personal life can free you from the toxic physical and emotional results of hanging on to these mistakes.

As a nurse, you understand the effects that constant activation of the sympathetic nervous system has on the body. Treating your emotional wounds is just as important as treating the physical ones you so vigilantly care for with your patients. Focusing on your past mistakes only gives energy to those internal wounds and keeps the story alive.

Instead, you can learn from your past and continue to make choices that support the vision for your highest self. You don't expect others to be flawless, and it's unrealistic to expect that of yourself either. So, give yourself the same understanding, compassion, and flexibility you would give to a close friend.

This emotional self-care activity will give you a quick and easy guide to practicing self-forgiveness. Grab a sheet of paper and write a list of three things you need to forgive yourself for. Take a few deep breaths and then acknowledge what you choose to forgive yourself for today. Then, for every statement on your list, write, "I forgive myself for [list item]. I free myself from it starting now."

After you've done the exercise for each statement on your list, it's time to get rid of the piece of paper to show symbolically how the mistake is now processed and out of your life. You can burn it safely, crumble it, or shred it. You can use this writing exercise again anytime a mistake happens. Don't allow mistakes to hold space in your mind and life—acknowledge them, learn from them, but be sure to forgive yourself and move on from them.

DEVELOP POSITIVE AFFIRMATIONS

Being a caretaker can be overwhelming and exhausting at times. You're endlessly interacting with people...patients, doctors, surgeons, scores of other healthcare providers and administrators, family members, and managers. The list can go on forever! These constant interactions with people are also laced with traumatic experiences, patients' many requests, and your own life problems. It's understandable if you feel like you have gigantic weights on your shoulders.

Hearing positive feedback (that well-deserved "Thank you" or "Great job today!") really helps that weight feel manageable, but nurses often don't get enough of it. But, that's okay—you don't need to wait to hear those things from someone else; you can tell yourself anytime, anywhere.

Positive affirmations are short statements that can give you the power to improve how you think and feel, thereby nourishing your emotional health. They are short, sweet, and to the point, but they are very powerful because they create a positive narrative that runs through your life.

Here are a few positive affirmations that can fit various scenarios in your life:

- My work as a nurse has purpose and transforms lives.
- If I stay positive and work hard, I can make anything happen.

- I am making a difference, and I find joy in knowing that.
- I am bright, resilient, and a dedicated student.
- I have all of the resources I need to get through this shift.
- I am doing my best to see the good in people, and that is enough.
- My only limit is my own mind.
- Today is a fresh start. I will set realistic expectations for myself, I will let go of things that are outside of my control, and I will love myself for who I am.
- I breathe in courage, and I exhale doubt.
- I am confident that I will pass this exam because I have prepared myself to the fullest.
- Today I will breathe, observe, and remain calm before I respond to others at work.
- It is healthy to care about my patients' needs and also my own.
- Today I choose to be the energy I wish to attract.
- I can start over, change my mind, try and fail, start late, have doubts, and still succeed in my nursing career.
- It is not my responsibility to make others happy.
- I am an amazing nurse! The opinions and judgments of others are irrelevant.
- I have the power of saying "no" without an explanation.
- I am powerful beyond measure.
- I am enough. I am an inspiration even though I am not perfect. I am grateful for the rewarding work that I do.
- I can be assertive and strong while still being loving and kind.

CUDDLE WITH YOUR PET

For years, hospitals have used pet therapy to promote healing for patients of all ages. Enjoying the company of a furry friend can reduce stress levels, lessen pain, and uplift spirits. Think of a time when you had a rough shift or a stressful day of errands, and walked in to a joyful pet waiting to greet you. It wipes all those negative feelings clean, right? Pets provide a sense of comfort and unconditional love that can't be replaced.

Physical affection from your fur baby is important for emotional self-care, so don't hesitate to carve out time to show your pet some love. Whether you own a cat, dog, or hamster, your pet holds so much value in your life. Nurses, just like patients in the hospital, can benefit tremendously from the company of a pet. Grab a few comfy blankets and cuddle up on the couch while you watch TV, or sit on the floor with them in your arms. Invite your pet to spend extra time with you even above and beyond your normal quality time. Allotting undivided attention for your animal is also beneficial for them. You are their entire world and they undoubtedly appreciate snuggles too. Use this time to reflect on the importance of unconditional love, pure innocence, and loyalty.

CULTIVATE
FRIENDSHIPS AT WORK

Nurses depend on each other to get through the shift...to help a patient to the bathroom while you give medications to another, or to draw important blood work while you speak to family members. A nurse's duties are never-ending, and strong teamwork in the workplace is a necessity. But what about for emotional health and support? Building strong relationships with coworkers that develop into friendships will help cultivate more support for one another in more ways than with nursing tasks. Having emotional support during your shift can positively influence your career as a nurse. The motivation that results from a friendly work environment can be a powerful tool for professional growth.

Make the effort to get to know your coworkers. Ask them about their interests and personal life, without being too assertive... you will get the vibe of who you will be able to cross the friendship barrier with. Having people whom you can vent to and also offer a different perspective to can make you more successful in your job. Fostering this friendliness among coworkers can help develop a stronger teamwork environment and also promote better patient outcomes. Patients feel the energy of the unit, and positive energy can help healing tremendously. Don't be afraid to dive a little deeper next time you're socializing with a coworker— you won't regret it!

SAY NO SOMETIMES

The nursing profession tends to glamorize being a compliant team player and rule follower. While this mindset can cultivate a great work environment, it can also have a negative effect on your self-care and work-life balance. Constantly agreeing to everything that is asked of you doesn't necessarily make you a good nurse—or a good partner, friend, or parent. If you are called on your day off and asked to work an overtime shift, but you'd rather stay home and recharge, it's okay to decline. When you're asked to take on an assignment that's beyond the scope of your skill set, it's okay to refuse and maybe help the person find another solution.

Shifting your priority to self-care and self-love will ultimately make you into a better nurse. Chances are, you're going above and beyond often enough anyway, so saying no sometimes is perfectly acceptable. You also don't need to apologize for every extra shift you can't take or any accommodation you can't make. Regularly saying sorry for things that don't require an apology or explanation can hinder your emotional well-being. Be confident in your choices.

Saying no might not come easily at first. Just like anything else, it may take some practice. It might help to brainstorm some phrases to have ready in your mind, such as these:

- My plate is too full to take that on.
- That won't work with my schedule.
- That's not my area of expertise.
- Thanks for asking, but I can't right now.

As you can see, you can still be kind in your response while you also honor your own emotional needs. If you need some time to prepare, tell the person you need to think about the request, then plan what you'll say in response. Saying no without guilt or apology is a great skill to carry with you in many areas of life.

FOLLOW YOUR INTUITION

"Nursing intuition" is a term we've been hearing since nursing school. There's no explanation for how you develop this intuition that allows you to quickly identify the needs and demands of a given situation or patient. Maybe it's something innate, or maybe it follows experience, thanks to a greater knowledge base and critical thinking. Regardless, it is vital that you recognize this instinct and trust that you should follow it. This intuition can help with minor situations and even huge ones, like when you follow your gut thinking that something is wrong and end up saving a patient's life. But it's easy to get lost in your many logistical tasks and focus more on structure than on listening to your intuition.

In order to start trusting these instincts, you'll need to practice finding stillness so you can listen to your inner voice. This stillness is challenging for nurses to find, when a million things are fighting for your attention and you're surrounded by noise, high stress, mixed emotions, and chaotic thoughts. Duck into a supply closet, go to the bathroom, or pop into a stairwell—grab a minute or two to stop and breathe so you can connect with your inner voice.

The more you practice this, the louder and stronger that inner voice becomes amid the daily noise. Eventually you might not need to be in near silence to hear it. Whenever you get a premonition about something during your shift, take a moment to recognize the feeling, reflect on evidence that can make it true, and pursue to take action. Believe in yourself!

CHAPTER TWO

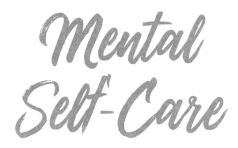
Mental Self-Care

Nursing comes with a myriad of responsibilities and duties that keep your body and mind busy. As soon as you wake up, the wheels start turning and everything from to-do lists and errands begins to pile up—and that's before you even get to work! There, you are expected to remember each patient's diagnoses, medical history, scheduled tests, medications, lab values, and so much more! It's completely understandable if your mind feels cluttered.

Practicing mental self-care will help you clear your mind and manage your stress. The self-care activities in this chapter are meant to help you form healthy habits at work, but many also apply in your everyday life as well. Carving out time to prioritize your mental well-being is important not only for yourself but for others around you—both your patients and loved ones. Regularly practicing mental self-care can help you maintain professionalism at work and healthy relationships with family and friends.

Many factors have a big impact on your mental health on a daily basis, such as the news, work emails, or scrolling through social media. That's why it is important that you are aware of the things around you that can have a negative impact on your mental state. Even something relatively small, like avoiding traffic during your work commute, can have you feeling like a different person. In this chapter, you will find self-care activities that will help you deal with small- and big-picture stressors. Activities like finding a therapist, using a stress ball, and trying breathing exercises to calm the mind will build awareness and inspire you to prioritize yourself.

LEARN SOMETHING NEW

Nurses certainly understand the value of knowledge. After all, a big part of your job is educating patients and families on tests, medications, procedures, and treatment plans.

Don't forget to turn the tables every once in a while and learn something new yourself, though! Learning a new skill helps create new neural pathways that can boost brain health. Nursing can take a lot from you mentally, physically, and emotionally, so choose something unrelated to this field. Step away from that world to recharge your mind and find pleasure in one of the numerous things there are to learn in the world.

Learning something new doesn't mean you have to enroll in an intense college-level course and spend months immersed in the topic. You might take a six-week pottery-throwing course at a local community center or watch a video online about how to plant a great vegetable garden in your yard. Maybe you've been meaning to pick up a new language—if so, you might be able to listen to lessons during your commute to work. Whatever you choose to do, make sure that it's not too much of a time commitment and that it's something you'll look forward to doing. This type of mental stimulation will keep your mind fresh and inspire you to keep learning throughout your life.

GO FOR A WALK
TO CLEAR YOUR MIND

Nurses focus so much energy and attention on educating patients on a healthy lifestyle. You talk about how vital it is to exercise and develop healthy eating habits. Be sure you take your own advice and fit short walks into your day whenever possible. They are beneficial not only for cardiovascular health but also for your mental health. Going for a walk with the intention to clear your mind is simple and effective, and doesn't require much time—even five or ten minutes can have a big impact.

Research shows that walking—especially outdoors—improves self-perception, mood, sleep quality, stress, and anxiety. If you are struggling to find time to walk, try carving out fifteen minutes in the morning or after dinner. If you want to walk during your work shift, try inviting a coworker to join you on your lunch break so you have some company. (Venting to someone is also a positive method to release pent-up stress!) But taking a walk on your own works just as well too.

As you walk, set a goal to focus on your breathing, the scenery you see, the feeling of fresh air, and the sounds around you. Think of positive affirmations (such as the ones from the Develop Positive Affirmations activity in Chapter 1) that you can recite in your head during your walk, and you'll soon start to notice how clear your mind becomes.

DO A JIGSAW PUZZLE

Whether you are a big fan of puzzles or haven't done one in years, you might be surprised to find out there are so many benefits to puzzle solving for adults. When you are solving puzzles, you strengthen the neurons in your brain, building stronger connections that help speed up your thought process. Enhancing this part of the brain allows you to recall bits and pieces of information that will form the big picture. The steps to finishing a jigsaw puzzle are actually pretty similar to how you process a problem at work. Nurses need to be creative and to think critically at all times. Working on a puzzle can also enhance your attention to detail, manage stress levels, encourage you to look for new perspectives, and improve your reasoning. Sounds like the perfect skill set for nursing!

Aside from all of the mental health points, puzzle solving is also fun! Choose a pretty picture of nature or a fun pop-culture image, or get a puzzle customized with a memorable family picture. Then make yourself a cup of tea and get puzzling.

"PAUSE FOR FIVE" WHEN YOU FEEL OVERWHELMED

When was the last time you felt stressed, overwhelmed, and unsure of what to do next at work? Those things happen so often, it was most likely during your last shift. Picture a to-do list that looks like this: Listen to new orders from the doctor, draw important labs for a patient, help a frail elderly patient in the bathroom, and coordinate a blood transfusion with another patient with low blood pressure. How do you prioritize among these patients? This creates both a moral and logistical dilemma for nurses because they are all important patients who need you in that moment.

Nurses get mentally and physically pulled in different directions all day long. Staying mentally clear and focused will help you face these difficult situations. It will be detrimental for you and your patient if you make a decision fueled by fear or anxiety. This activity will help you declutter your mind, leaving you with the ability to process your tasks and organize your priorities. (This is also a strategy you can take with you outside of work!) It requires no equipment and takes only seconds to do.

This is called the "Pause for Five" technique. It's a way for you to get away from the hustle and bustle for just a brief moment.

Even in the midst of the chaos around you, you always have the power to clear your mind in order to be a more efficient nurse. Here's how:

1. Take a quick moment to pause. If you feel comfortable, close your eyes.
2. Take a few deep breaths, in and out, as you slowly count to five in your head.
3. Feel free to say (aloud or silently) a positive affirmation or picture peaceful scenery.
4. Allow your mind to clear and free up space for a solution.
5. Observe your heart rate slow down as you breathe.

As you reopen your eyes and return to your regular breathing, you will likely find yourself better able to assess what's in front of you and sort out what's most urgent.

PLAN A FEW HOURS
OF ALONE TIME

Apart from dealing with patients all day, you are constantly communicating with and in the presence of coworkers. The list of people you come in contact with every shift is endless. Though this teamwork is part of what makes the medical field so successful, it can also be mentally draining. Planning a few hours of alone time will help you reconnect with yourself and recharge your batteries.

What you do with this time is completely up to you. The goal of this activity is for you to focus on yourself. There's a wonderful sense of freedom that comes with enjoying your own company, but you might not have experienced it in ages. Take this time to unapologetically and selfishly attend to your own interests. Use the few hours to go shopping and then treat yourself to lunch. Or simply take a nap. Getting extra sleep might be a rare occurrence for you, so relish it!

After you enjoy one of these sessions, you will probably find yourself eager to plan another one. When you're alone you have the power to really think about how you feel, without anyone else's input. This feeling shouldn't be a luxury, but rather something you enjoy regularly!

USE A STRESS BALL

Stress is all around you in your professional, social, and personal life. You've probably got an endless to-do list at work, but your responsibilities don't end there—you also have a list of things waiting for you at home. Sometimes a simple, easy way to relieve stress might be just the ticket to get you through a shift or day.

Enter the squishy stress ball! Keeping a small stress ball in your scrub pocket, work bag, car, or locker is an easy way to make sure you get relief whenever you need it most. These balls come in various shapes and sizes, so look for one that fits comfortably in the palm of your hand. You can pull it out whenever you need to release a little tension.

Squeezing the ball activates your wrist and hand muscles, and releasing the grip relaxes them. This motion helps alleviate stress and tension, which nurses carry so much of. The stress ball can help you relax *and* strengthen your hand muscles, which you use all the time to document everything!

TRY MEDITATION

Has someone ever told you to "just relax" when you're in the middle of a stressful situation, and you can't help but think, "That's easy for you to say!"? The ability to relax doesn't come naturally for most people. It's difficult not to get consumed in worry, whether it is from a demanding job, financial hardship, hectic life, or lack of time with friends and family.

The good news is that you can teach yourself to relax. One strategy is by learning how to meditate. Think of meditation as a simple way to improve your overall mental health and well-being. It doesn't have to mean sitting cross-legged on a remote mountain—meditation can be done in lots of easy ways almost anytime, anywhere. Meditation has many potential benefits, including reducing anxiety and tension, improving sleep quality, minimizing memory loss, and decreasing blood pressure. Plus, when you're in a stressful situation, fight-or-flight hormones are released that cause your heart rate to increase, your muscles to tense up, and your breathing to intensify. Meditation will provide you with the proper skills in order to control this response whenever you need.

To get started, try this simple ten-minute gratitude meditation:

1. Get into a comfortable position, lying down or sitting with your hands softly in your lap.
2. Sit up tall, elongating your spine. Close your eyes and bring all of your awareness to your breath.
3. Notice how your breath flows in and out. When you breathe in, your belly should expand while your rib cage lengthens.

4. As you exhale, release the negative energy you've been building up.
5. Think about how grateful you are to breathe in and out, and to be where you are right now.
6. Appreciate your lungs for allowing you to breathe, and your heart and brain for keeping you alive.
7. Continue to focus on your breath, allowing thoughts to come and go.

At first, it can be difficult to keep your mind clear, but it's okay if you find thoughts arising while you breathe. When that happens, simply acknowledge the thought, then let it go. Be flexible and gentle with yourself as you learn. Start with shorter amounts of time, such as ten minutes, and build up to twenty or thirty as you get more practice. Do your best to meditate regularly so you get frequent practice.

If you find you like the experience, you may even want to dedicate a space in your home where you can cultivate tranquil and peaceful vibes. Lay down a yoga mat and a comfy pillow, and place a plant and maybe a candle nearby. If you'd like to vary up your meditation, look for guided meditations that you can listen to online or from an app. It can take a little practice for meditation to feel comfortable and easy, but it's worth the time and effort to experience true relaxation and a clear mind.

ENJOY AROMATHERAPY

Sometimes taking a mental break can be as simple as sitting down and relaxing by one of your favorite scented candles, essential oil diffusers, or incense sticks. Aromatherapy can reduce stress, improve your quality of sleep, and encourage relaxation. Plus, it's inexpensive and easy to incorporate into your day.

Keep a few options stocked in your home, with various scents, so you're always prepared for any type of mood. Here are a few examples:

- When you're having trouble calming your mind or need help relaxing before bed, try scents like lavender, chamomile, or rose.
- For something more energizing, try citrus or mint scents.
- To boost your immune system, try cinnamon or eucalyptus.
- Always make sure you extinguish anything lighted before you doze off. If you find this activity beneficial, share the love and gift a scented candle to a coworker who has been having rough shifts!

LOSE YOURSELF IN ANOTHER WORLD WITH A BOOK

Finding time in your day to sit back and relax can be challenging for nurses—your mind and body are always on the go. Even when you're not on duty you have things that need to be checked off the to-do list. Just like getting laundry done, though, you should schedule in mental self-care and relaxation as part of the day.

To do that, there's nothing like getting lost in a good book. It can take your mind to a different world, far away from your responsibilities and worries. You're able to put yourself in someone else's shoes—maybe even in a different time and place. Plus, reading quiets your mind, boosts your mood, inspires creativity, and improves cognitive function. The positive changes in the brain caused by reading continue even after you put the book down! Long-term effects of this mental exercise are similar to meditation, activating an inner calm every nurse needs.

Whether you're into romance, mystery, or science fiction, choose something you can enjoy. Try to read for at least thirty minutes several times a week. If you want to add a social component, read the same book as a friend and discuss it afterward. Or, join a low-stress local book club.

FIND A THERAPIST

It is no secret that nurses deal with the type of trauma that can lead to bouts of sadness or even depression. There are shifts that make you want to curl up in a ball and cry, or run out of the room screaming with frustration. But no matter what, you probably suck it up and persevere. Nurses don't break down; they get used to it, right? No.

This misguided mentality can eventually lead to serious anxiety and depression without your even being aware of it. That's why finding a professional therapist is a smart idea for nurses. Therapy is a way for you to understand certain emotions, reflect on traumatic shifts, discover solutions to conflict, learn new things about yourself, and even develop tactics to cope with stress. Not only will it be beneficial for your professional life, but it will also improve your personal life.

Don't be afraid to take your time when finding the right therapist. One place to start is by checking with your insurance to see if they can give you a list of therapists in your area that are covered under your plan. Do some background research on the options to see what they value and the theories they use in their practice. If you and a therapist don't have the right chemistry, move on to someone with a different style. It's important to find the right connection for optimal results. Some therapists offer virtual meetings along with in-person, which might be beneficial with your busy schedule.

You don't need to have a major crisis to see a therapist—think of it as an investment in your mental health just as a gym membership is an investment in your physical health. Try working sessions into your weekly or monthly calendar so you have regularly scheduled check-ins.

DELETE APPS/GAMES
THAT DRAIN YOU

Dealing with patients, doctors, families, and managers all day can be demanding. Sometimes you just need some time away from interacting with people, so you turn to your phone. While scrolling through TikTok periodically might be entertaining and positive for mental self-care, overconsumption can be harmful. App developers design their apps to promote addiction, so don't feel bad if you have lost a lot of time to a brightly colored game.

Perhaps you can relate to how overconsumption of cell phone use affects your relationships, reduces your work efficiency, and leaves you less likely to have real conversations with people. Exhausting your mental supply on apps can also leave you feeling foggy.

To break out of this habit, delete the apps that usually consume lots of time and leave you feeling empty. You'll probably miss the app at first but then forget all about it. When you find yourself reaching for your phone to play a game, try doing an activity from this book instead. This cleansing process will ultimately save you the time and energy you need to get other things done!

ENJOY A SKIN TREATMENT AT A SPA

Though stress is affiliated with your mental state, it's also something you carry with you physically. Muscle tension, headaches, and stomachaches are just some of the aches and pains that can be attributed to stress. Beyond those, you may also notice minor skin issues, like acne breakouts, rashes, and redness. Your skin probably takes a lot of abuse as a nurse—you're washing your hands frequently, wearing masks a lot, and on your feet all day long. Why not take time out to pamper your skin with a spa treatment?

The range of services offered at spas nowadays is so vast! Whether you want a traditional facial or mani-pedi or something different, like a cryofacial, cupping, or a mud bath, there's something for every skin type and personality. (And remember, spas are not just for women!) If you're having trouble finding a spa near you, see if an upscale hotel that's nearby has one that non-guests can visit.

Just as you would schedule a dentist appointment, make time to treat your skin with the care it deserves. Sit back, relax, and let someone else take care of you for a change!

USE BREATHING EXERCISES TO CALM YOUR MIND

Have you ever noticed how different your breathing pattern is when you're relaxed? When your mind is calm (like when you're about to fall asleep or taking a bubble bath), you breathe deeper and slower, with a more regular and controlled rhythm. When you're stressed, your breathing is more shallow and irregular. Luckily, you can teach yourself to reclaim a controlled breathing style even in stressful situations by practicing breathing exercises.

There are many different breathing exercises that you can incorporate into your daily routine to help calm your mind. The greatest part about this activity is that you can do them anywhere: while you're on your lunch break, during an emergency situation, while you're confronting a coworker, or even when you're dealing with a noncompliant patient. As you're first learning them, however, try to practice when you are calm and can focus completely on your body. Then, once you get comfortable with the techniques, incorporate them anytime you need.

4-7-8 BREATHING

1. Take a deep breath in through your nose while counting to 4.
2. Gently hold the breath and count to 7.
3. Exhale through your mouth completely as you count to 8.
4. Repeat 3 to 5 times until you feel relaxed.

BELLY BREATHING

1. Place one hand on your belly and another on your chest.
2. Slowly inhale through your nose and notice how your belly rises but your chest remains still.
3. Exhale using pursed lips as you tighten your core muscles.
4. Focus on the belly rise and fall for 8 to 10 breaths.

EQUAL BREATHING

1. Count to 5 as you inhale deeply.
2. Exhale while you count to 5.
3. Note: Instead of counting to 5, you can choose a word to repeat with each inhale and exhale, making sure your breaths are equal in duration.

No matter which breathing method works best for you, they all help you concentrate on your inhale and exhale in order to relax, reduce muscle tension, and relieve stress. The way you breathe affects your entire body, and in high-stress situations you want to be as in control of your body as possible. (Pro tip: Breathing exercises can even help you fall asleep quicker!) Tuning in to your breathing will come in handy both at work and in your personal life.

HANG UP AN INSPIRATIONAL QUOTE

Words hold the power to heal, inspire, and rejuvenate you. Whether it's reading a calming quote when you're stressed, a funny quote when you're down, or a motivational quote when you're feeling discouraged, words of encouragement can really turn your day around. You can ensure that you always have words of wisdom around you if you hang up an important quote or two in your home or workstation.

There are many ways to find quotes that resonate with you. It can be as simple as doing a Google search, downloading an app that sends you uplifting thoughts daily, or following inspirational accounts on social media. Here are some ideas to get you started:

- "A ship is safe in harbor, but that is not what ships are built for."
  —John A. Shedd

- "Never be limited by other people's limited imaginations."
  —Mae Jemison

- "Don't spend time beating on a wall, hoping to transform it into a door."
  —Coco Chanel

- "No one can make you feel inferior without your consent."
  —Eleanor Roosevelt

- "You are your best thing."
  —Toni Morrison

Once you find some quotes that you really understand and connect with, print and frame them. Hang them up in a place where you'll see them frequently so they can provide a positive mental boost whenever you need one.

START A DAILY JOURNAL

Making lists, documenting assessments, and writing notes to the providers are all things that nurses do without even thinking twice. But how often do you write down your own thoughts, hopes, and dreams? Journaling can help organize your thoughts while helping reduce stress and anxiety. Maybe the best part of journaling is how flexible it is. You can write one line a day or three pages; you can write in a lovely bound notebook or on your phone; you can write first thing in the morning or before you go to bed. Making journaling a part of your daily routine can help you heal from some of the trauma you witness on the job by working through emotions that might be buried deep in your mind.

A simple "everyday method" you can use is writing about your day, start to finish. Jot down the events, your emotions, any accomplishments, what you could've done differently, and so on. If that method doesn't appeal to you, consider using one of these prompts:

- Write down three memories that make you smile.
- Write a love letter to yourself.

- When you are feeling stressed or overwhelmed, write how you physically feel from head to toe.
- Finish the statement "I am strong because..."
- Think about this statement: "Something I want to learn more about is...because..."
- What happened in a good dream you had, and how did it make you feel?
- In which area of your life can you practice more patience?

The more you know about your thoughts, the more active a role you can play in understanding them. You will be able to identify regular thought patterns and behaviors that trigger stress and anxiety for you. And in turn, you can then come up with solutions on how to improve. Journaling is also an opportunity for positive self-talk.

Journaling is a powerful tool for self-discovery and personal development and for giving all that chatter in your head somewhere to go. Experiment to see what methods and times work best for you, then try to work it into your daily schedule.

ALIGN YOUR SOCIAL MEDIA USAGE WITH YOUR MENTAL WELL-BEING

There's no doubt about it: Your social media habits can affect your mood. Though you may feel like you scroll through feeds mindlessly, it's not actually a mindless activity. Everything you are exposed to subconsciously shifts your mood, thoughts, and perspective. Plus, most people inevitably start to compare themselves to other people—and usually in a negative light (for example, wondering why your body can't look like that person's, or why that other friend always seems to be able to go on vacations and you can't). These comparisons can be detrimental to your mental well-being.

Regain control of what you see by doing a deep cleanse on who you follow. Set aside an hour, think about how this process can improve your mental well-being, and unfollow or mute anyone whose posts make you feel bad. Make sure the accounts you follow are encouraging and align with your interests, values, and goals. (Pro tip: There are also many great nursing accounts that provide self-care tips, nurse hacks, clinical information, and study tools!)

Once you've gone through your list, see if you can start to follow any new accounts that could lift your mood and enhance your life. You may notice that your experience with social media leads to many fewer negative comparisons and many more boosts in energy and positivity!

PLAN AN ADVENTURE

Nursing can be very adventurous, but this activity is for a different a kind of adrenaline rush! If you've been feeling a little down or bored by your routine, try planning an adventure. Challenge yourself to push the envelope and do something fun and exciting to get you out of that mental rut. Stepping out of the norm will elevate your mood, give you mental clarity, and celebrate your true self.

What you do and who you do it with is completely up to you. The choices are endless. An outdoor adventure like hiking, rock climbing, zip lining, stand-up paddleboarding, or horseback riding will bring you closer to nature and ground your soul. You can also find plenty of indoor options that can provide a thrill, like going to an escape room, getting a tattoo, singing karaoke at a new bar, throwing axes, or playing laser tag. If you want to try something bolder and have the time and budget, travel to a new country.

Once you've decided what you want to do, choose a date and commit to it. If you want to get a bit of advance knowledge, read forums or reviews about this activity so you can check out other people's recommendations. No matter what you choose, get ready to feel mentally restored and energized after you do it!

PICK UP A CREATIVE HOBBY

The nursing profession requires you to be instinctive and creative on a daily basis. Whether you realize it or not, you come up with innovative solutions for unique patient situations all the time. How many times have you figured out different ways to use a piece of equipment? Or maybe you've created something that makes your work life easier with the supplies you have in your utility closet. Nurses are always thinking of ways to improve and get things done more efficiently. Starting a creative hobby can allow you to use all of those inventive skills in a totally different way.

A good hobby can be entertaining and fulfilling, both of which are important for mental self-care. Picking up a creative hobby can be exciting and rewarding because you're crafting something yourself. Creative hobbies aren't just limited to drawing and painting, either. Here are some other ideas to get you started:

- Sewing
- Gardening
- Jewelry making
- Photography/scrapbooking
- Furniture restoration
- Knitting

Make sure to give yourself a good chunk of time to complete your project and avoid interruptions if possible. Don't worry too much about the finished product—it doesn't have to be perfect. What's key is that you are taking your mind off work and sparking your creative energy. You can keep, gift, or sell your creation when you're done!

CHAPTER THREE

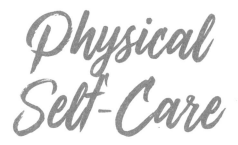

Physical Self-Care

You likely spend hours educating your patients on how to take care of their bodies: the importance of a healthy diet and an ideal sleep schedule, proper body alignment, taking breaks to avoid burnout, getting preventative medical tests, and so on. But when was the last time you followed your own recommendations? Taking care of your own body is something you might ignore or at least put on the back burner. After all, a nurse's mind is wired from the first day of nursing school to put the patient first. Yet the goal of nursing is not to wear you down. There is no prize for the most overworked and exhausted nurse.

It's time to turn the tables and examine how you're taking care of your own body. How much physical activity are you doing? How is your quality of sleep? What kinds of foods are you fueling your body with? How are you protecting yourself and preventing injuries? Nurses are regularly lifting and turning patients, on their feet for most of their shifts, and tirelessly walking from room to room. All of these things require an enormous amount of physical energy! In this chapter, you will find activities that will help optimize and fuel that energy. For example, you'll learn how to start an exercise routine, meal prep for your shifts, make a nutritious smoothie, wear the right shoes at work, and reduce your sugar intake.

Being aware of ways to improve your own physical self-care will also expand the knowledge you can share with your patients and coworkers. Even when it seems difficult, try to make time for these physical self-care activities on a regular basis. You will realize the difference a healthy body makes in how you function, both during your shifts and after them!

TAKE A HOT BUBBLE BATH

This activity is a great choice after a long day of work. You know—the kind of shift where you didn't sit once, maybe took a short break, and felt pulled in every direction at once. You probably feel like your mind, body, and soul were all dragged across concrete. A hot bubble bath is not only emotionally therapeutic, but also perfect for soothing sore muscles. A hot bath also allows the time and space for you to breathe deeper and slower, promoting stress relief.

There's no wrong way to take a bubble bath, but here are some helpful tips. If you are sweaty or dirty, you might want to take a quick shower before your bath. Then, get the temperature just right—you want it warm enough to feel soothing but not *too* hot. Bubble baths with soothing scents like lavender might be a good choice for a relaxing bath. If bubbles aren't your thing, consider adding Epsom salts, which can aid in muscle swelling and joint inflammation. If scented bath products irritate your skin, try diffusing essential oils, like lavender, nearby for relaxing vibes. Lie back and let the warm, peaceful water wash away your tension and aches.

PLAN HEALTHY WORK SNACKS IN ADVANCE

Nursing is physically taxing, so you've got to fuel your body to make it through a shift. Often, though, the easiest snacks to grab quickly are unhealthy options from vending machines or cafeterias. Instead of relying on those choices, prepare and bring your own healthy snacks so you can give your body essential vitamins and minerals instead of a lot of fat and empty calories.

Healthy snacks don't have to be tasteless! Plan your favorites in different categories like salty, sweet, and savory so you're prepared for any craving. For example, stress can evoke the need for salty foods, and it's so tempting to want potato chips or fries. Instead, try bringing small bags of these healthier options:

- Almonds or cashews
- Hard-boiled eggs with everything seasoning
- Pretzels
- Popcorn
- Kale chips
- Olives
- Baked carrot chips
- Edamame with sea salt

Craving something sweet? Don't worry—you can still appease your sweet tooth while giving your body nutrients. Feed your belly and brain with snacks like these:

- Dark chocolate
- Greek yogurt with berries
- Fruit salad
- Protein bars
- Sliced apples with peanut butter
- Dates
- Homemade trail mix with dried fruit or dark chocolate chips

When preparing your snacks, make sure they're nutritious, simple, and filling. If you need more ideas, look on *Pinterest* or other social media sites. It might take a few minutes to prepare the snacks, but you'll be thanking yourself later when you're starving mid-shift. These healthy snacks will help you get rid of those hunger pains while simultaneously increasing your energy level, improving your brain function, and enhancing your work performance.

SHUT OFF SCREENS
BEFORE BED

Quality sleep is a necessity for nurses, but getting the proper amount of shut-eye can be challenging.

While it can improve life in so many ways, technology can prevent your mind from relaxing. Plus, chances are you're not doing anything strictly necessary—you're probably scrolling through social media or playing a game while lying in bed. You might be accustomed to mindlessly relying on your phone, tablet, or TV to escape from a stressful day, but then you lose track of time and stay up way past your bedtime. (Yes, adults need a *bedtime*.)

Why is blue light from screens so concerning? It disturbs the natural production of melatonin, a hormone that aids in sleep. You pay the price by throwing off your circadian rhythm, making it harder to fall asleep.

One way you set yourself up for a good night's sleep is by creating a "no screen time" policy that begins thirty minutes before your bedtime. (Screen time includes TVs, cell phones, tablets, computers, and laptops...basically anything that emits blue light.) Instead of screen time, try meditating or reading a book in bed. This will help quiet your thoughts and let your body naturally get ready for some much-needed z's.

STAY HYDRATED WITH A FUN WATER BOTTLE

Getting the right amount of daily water intake is difficult, especially for nurses. Since you're rarely in one place for long, it can be difficult to keep yourself hydrated. Still, proper hydration is key to maintaining optimal physical health, so if you're not drinking enough water, it's time to get creative.

One simple and motivating way to stay on top of your water intake is by using a fun water jug. The daily recommendation for water intake is about two liters, so getting a bottle this size would be ideal. Find a bottle that fits your personality in terms of color and style and has a convenient spout. If you find yourself going long periods without drinking, buy a jug with timed reminders labeled every few ounces. This will hold you accountable for when that time comes even on your busiest shifts!

In order for your body to perform at its optimal level, it has to be properly hydrated. Water helps get rid of toxins, lubricates your joints, protects your organs, and allows for temperature regulation. You will also reap additional benefits, like increased energy levels, improved brain function, and enhanced focus.

START AN EXERCISE ROUTINE

You know you should exercise...but finding the time, energy, or motivation can be a challenge. One way to overcome that hurdle is by figuring out a routine that will work for you. By making exercise a regular part of your routine, you earn all of the beneficial cardiovascular effects, weight loss, immune system support, blood pressure control, and so much more.

You may need to do a little trial and error to sort out when you can fit in exercise based on what your body needs. For example, jogging before your shift can be a great pick-me-up to get you ready and motivated for a busy day, while boxing after work can be a great way to release some built-up stress. If you're just getting started with your exercise journey, start off with short workouts and build yourself up to longer ones as you boost your stamina. Remember that exercise can be fun! Try a dance workout with a friend if you like energetic, social workouts. If you prefer solo exercise, consider a long bike ride. There are also many workouts you can find online and on apps that make it easy to exercise at home or inside in any weather.

Here are some ideas you might find helpful as you create an exercise routine:

- **Shoes:** Go to a local sporting goods store and get fitted for sneakers that match your activity. The coolest-looking ones might not offer the right support level for your feet or gait, so keep an open mind and prioritize comfort over fashion.

- **Water:** Make sure you have water accessible to you as you exercise. You may want to look for water with electrolytes to help balance your system.
- **Headphones:** Good music is always a great motivational tool to get you in the right headspace for an impactful workout. Invest in earbuds or headphones that are made for movement and activity. If you are exercising around town, be sure you can still hear your surroundings so you stay aware and safe.
- **Proper attire:** Whether you find comfort in shorts or long spandex pants, find the right fit and fabric to avoid chafing. Wear undergarments that are supportive and comfortable.
- **Fitness tracker:** You can find a variety of fitness trackers on the market that capture your steps, heart rate, and other exercise data. The prices and quality range, so choose whatever fits your lifestyle.

Exercise is not only a great way to maintain physical health; it can also impact your mental health! Working out can control stress and boost the body's ability to deal with mental fatigue. While you are getting your heart rate up, your body releases endorphins, which provide you with a wide range of benefits like improved memory and focus, better multitasking abilities, elevated mood, antidepressive effects, and sharper information recall. So get exercising and reap those rewards!

TRY A NEW RECIPE

Everyone has staple recipes they make frequently, and there is no shame in that! But sometimes you need to change things up and try a new recipe—one with unique flavors or ingredients you haven't tried before is a great choice.

You can involve your partner or family in this activity too. Everyone can choose a new recipe to try, and/or you can all help prepare the food. To boost the nutritional value, follow the US Department of Agriculture's MyPlate guidelines and try to eat fruits and vegetables, whole grains, and high-quality protein alongside a small amount of dairy. Visit www.myplate.gov/myplate-kitchen to find healthy recipes you and your family might enjoy.

Making a new recipe can help refresh your weekly menu options and boost your vitamin and mineral intake—and you might just find a dish that becomes a new favorite!

TAKE VITAMINS AND SUPPLEMENTS

Do you wake up some days feeling fatigued, sick, or mentally fogged and don't really know why? It might be because you're lacking essential nutrients.

Many of your daily nutrient requirements can be fulfilled with your food intake, but that depends on how vigilant you are with your diet. Nurses are on a time constraint as it is, juggling long shifts and everything else in their personal life. Calculating your daily vitamin and mineral intake shouldn't be a part of the daily stress. A simple way to fill the gaps in your diet and ensure your body is getting the appropriate amount of nutrients is by taking dietary supplements.

So where do you begin? First, contact your medical provider to be sure you're taking a mixture that's right for you. In all likelihood, a multivitamin is a safe bet. These come in both liquid and pill form, and sometimes as gummies. Other basic supplements to consider are calcium, omega-3 fatty acids, iron, probiotics, and vitamins B, C, and D. Benefits of proper vitamin intake include supporting bone health, preventing cell damage, improving brain function, aiding with sleep, keeping organs functioning properly, and revitalizing physical energy.

TREAT YOURSELF TO A MASSAGE

Raise your hand if your body feels tense, achy, and dragged down after a stretch of long shifts! Your body exerts a vast amount of physical energy between constantly moving patients in and out of bed and walking quickly to and from the medication room. Having a job that keeps you active is good for your overall health, but you also have to be sure you're pampering yourself once in a while too. A massage is a great way to do that.

In fact, a massage is just as important for your muscles as sticking to your workout routine and practicing good posture because a massage will break down hardened and constricted fascia (which are those knots you always get in your neck or back). Common complaints that are caused by fascia are sciatic pain, headaches, and neck pain.

Some other benefits of massage include reduced stress, relief from muscle pain, and improved sleep (thanks to the pain relief and stress reduction). Better sleep, less pain, and relaxation? That's music to a nurse's ear.

Massages can easily feel like an unaffordable luxury, but there are many options to choose from. Here are just a few:

- If you want all the bells and whistles, start with a full-body massage at a professional spa (maybe you can ask for it as a gift when your birthday rolls around).
- For a more affordable and time-friendly choice, try a ten-minute back massage at a local nail salon.
- Another recommendation is to use a company that sends massage therapists to your home, if your priorities are privacy and convenience.

Don't forget to check your medical insurance to see if it covers any massages. Some wellness centers offer massage therapy and accept insurance as a form of payment.

MAKE A NUTRITIOUS SMOOTHIE

You know you need lots of vitamins and minerals to maintain a healthy body. But finding time and recipes to incorporate each one into your diet can be time-consuming. Instead, try smoothies—they are a simple and easy way to make a nutrient-packed meal you can even take on the go.

If you like to experiment with flavors, search online for recipes that look tasty. These ideas might help get you started:

- A basic green smoothie recipe includes almond milk (or water), spinach, kale, pineapple, and avocado.
- If you're looking for extra protein, try using almond milk, banana, protein powder, frozen berries, and peanut butter.
- Of course there are many variations of fruits, milk, seeds, supplements, and vegetables you can add.
- If trial and error isn't your thing, consider store-bought or premade options. Some companies will even deliver premade smoothie packets right to your door! If you buy smoothies, keep an eye on the nutritional panel to be sure there isn't too much added sugar.

Whether you sip your smoothie on the way to work, during your break, or on your off days, your body and mind will thank you for the nutritional boost!

PRACTICE YOGA
TO RELIEVE STRESS

The stress that nursing brings into your life can be taxing on your body and your mind. Finding coping mechanisms that deal with stress in positive ways is vital for your physical well-being. Yoga is a great tool to help combat all of the negative effects that stress can have on your body.

Yoga is a practice that combines physical poses, controlled breathing, and meditation to sync your mind and body. You will gain improved balance, flexibility, range of motion, and strength, plus find yourself more relaxed and calm—and with a minimal amount of equipment! Some types of yoga, such as Hatha, Vinyasa, Bikram, and Ashtanga, are more geared toward fighting stress and finding serenity than others.

You can also do a quick yoga session as a part of your pre- or post-shift routine. Create your own short routine by choosing a few simple poses that you can do in the comfort of your own home. Try one of these options: Chair Pose, Cat/Cow Pose, Cobra, Child's Pose, Downward-Facing Dog, Mountain Pose, Seated Spinal Twist, Standing Forward Bend, Warrior 1, Warrior 2, and Triangle Pose. Look online for instructional videos and check your positioning in a mirror to be sure you're doing the poses correctly.

PROTECT YOUR BACK
WITH SAFE PATIENT HANDLING

Proper patient handling and body mechanics is vital in the nursing profession. You are frequently called upon to provide support, bear extra weight, and reach in difficult ways. Even though we've all watched the videos and taken the classes on proper posture and body mechanics, getting your patients comfortable takes priority in that moment and you might forget your training when you're crunched for time. Unfortunately, overexertion, repetitive bending and twisting, and excessive physical effort are only a few of the reasons why nurses suffer from various musculoskeletal injuries.

Safe patient handling involves the use of mechanical equipment, team lifts, and proper body techniques in order to assist patients without causing yourself harm. Protecting your back is of highest importance in these situations, regardless of patient size or medical condition. There are many ways for nurses to protect their bodies at work, such as these:

- Don't do everything alone. Ask for a coworker's help when needed—remember that nursing is a team effort. Sharing the load, even when using mechanical equipment, will reduce the strain on your body. There's no need to be the hero in these situations. If a patient requires more assistance than you can provide yourself, don't be afraid to get help.
- Keep the patient as close to you as possible to avoid over-reaching or overextending.

- Assess the need for mechanical equipment. If the patient isn't able to bear weight or stand appropriately with team lift, opt for mechanical transfer aids. Devices like the Hoyer lift, transfer boards, gait belts with handles, and sit-to-stand lifts require time but are highly beneficial.
- Know that injuries are not often from a single event. The repetitive movement of bending over the wrong way, not pushing from your legs, or forgetting to raise the bed for a turn can be just as detrimental over time. Take the extra time to do it right—every time. Remember all of the fundamental steps you learned and make them habits:
  - Raise the bed to hip level or where it's comfortable for you to boost and turn the patient. Never lean over the bed or kneel on the bed when transferring a patient.
  - Use a straight back and push from your legs when lifting. Don't forget to activate your core muscles and maintain a wide stance as well. This will protect you from spine strain.
- If you do suffer an injury, report it as soon as possible to protect yourself from further harm. Don't neglect it and continue your shift in the hope that the pain will go away.

If you make safer choices and remain consistent in your practices, they will quickly become habitual. If you're ever tempted to cut corners, remind yourself that if you hurt your back only to save a few minutes, you won't be well equipped to be anyone's nurse!

SIT DOWN WHILE
YOU DOCUMENT

It's difficult for nurses to sit down on the job due to the nature of your responsibilities. But you might not realize how straining it is on your joints, ligaments, and muscles when you stand for such long periods of time. The aches and pains that come as a result will show up eventually—either right away or just when you're comfy in bed trying to sleep. Try to find a few minutes here and there to sit during your shift—such as while you're catching up on paperwork and documentation—to rest your body. If you work in a very fast-paced environment, try sitting in small increments of five minutes every hour. You can still reap the benefits from little bursts of rest throughout your shift.

Remember: Grabbing a chair and resting your lower body doesn't make you any less of a nurse. Documenting is a major chunk of the nursing profession, so you might as well be comfortable while doing it. Maintaining good posture while sitting is also essential, so refer to the Practice Good Posture activity in this chapter for helpful tips. Sitting while you document can also help you improve your focus, increase your productivity and creativity, and preserve your energy for patient care. Your muscles work hard; they deserve a break!

TREAT YOURSELF
TO SOMETHING SWEET

Sure, most of the time you want to eat healthy fruits and vegetables that help you fuel your body for your taxing job and busy personal life. But every once in a while, you deserve a guilt-free sweet treat too!

Along with the fact that they taste great to most people, desserts elicit a chemical response from regions of the brain that control feelings of pleasure and reward—sugar and carbohydrates are linked with mood improvement and positive emotions.

If you're trying to stick closely to a diet or healthy eating lifestyle, you don't have to go way off track to enjoy something. Sweet treats can have healthy components too! Options like fruit salad, carrot cake, dark chocolate, frozen yogurt topped with granola and fruit, oatmeal raisin cookies, chocolate-covered almonds, an acai bowl, cheese and honey, frozen fruit pops, applesauce, or roasted honey-cinnamon peaches taste great but also offer nutritional benefits. Whatever you choose, savor it and remind yourself that you've earned this with all your hard work.

PRACTICE GOOD POSTURE

After the last long shift you worked, was your back aching, were your legs throbbing, or was your neck on fire? A lot of those aches and pains were likely due to poor posture. Whether you're sitting at a computer charting, standing while reviewing orders, or bending over adjusting a patient's pillow, good posture is key to physical self-care. Following are some easy ways you can practice good posture at work:

WHEN STANDING:

- Stand up straight and tall with your shoulders back.
- Pull in your core muscles.
- Bear most of your weight on the balls of your feet.
- Maintain a slight bend in your knees.
- Keep your head level; don't push your head forward.
- Keep your feet about shoulder-width apart.
- Shift your weight when needed if you're standing for a long time.

WHEN SITTING:

- Keep your feet on the ground without crossing your legs.
- Keep your knees at the same level as your hips.
- Relax your shoulders and keep them back.
- Adjust the back of your seat to support your mid- and lower back.
- Avoid sitting in the same position for long periods of time.

Incorrect alignment and posture can put significant strain on your joints and muscles and can ultimately lead to increased pain and even a chance of debilitating injuries. Utilizing proper strategies can help prevent these issues.

PLAN YOUR CAFFEINE INTAKE FOR THE DAY

Caffeine is a nurse's best friend. When you need to stay up for the night shift or get up early for the day shift, there's nothing better than that first sip to feel the rush of energy that will prepare you for the shift ahead. Whether you prefer coffee, tea, energy drinks, or soda, caffeine is a quick and effective stimulant, providing you with the perfect energy jolt whenever you need one. Moderate levels of caffeine intake have also been shown to improve memory, increase stamina, and boost metabolism. However, too much caffeine intake does have some fairly serious downsides. For example, it can cause anxiety, insomnia, heart palpitations, frequent urination, high blood pressure, dehydration, and even addiction.

You don't necessarily have to avoid caffeine entirely, but it is a good idea to know how much you're consuming. Planning out your daily caffeine intake will make you more aware of the amount you're drinking and set you on a schedule that could ultimately improve your sleep. The US Food and Drug Administration recommends no more than 400 milligrams of caffeine a day for most adults.

For reference, here's how much caffeine is in some popular drinks:

- 1 cup decaffeinated coffee or tea: 5–10 mg
- 1 cup green tea: 15–30 mg
- 1 (12-ounce) can cola: 40–50 mg
- 1 cup black tea: 60–75 mg
- 1 (12-ounce) can Red Bull: 110 mg
- 1 (12-ounce) cup coffee: 130–140 mg

To track your intake, plan out how much caffeine you're going to consume and when. It's easy to overconsume during a busy shift, so thinking about it ahead of time is worth the effort. For example, if you plan to have two cups of coffee at the start of your shift and some soda halfway through it, you'll know you probably shouldn't have too much more caffeine after that.

After you plan out your day, check to see that your last caffeine fix happens no less than six hours before your bedtime. This will allow your body to align with its natural circadian rhythm to optimize sleep. If you're craving the taste of your favorite drink but could go without the caffeine buzz, opt for the decaf version. Monitoring your caffeine intake will become second nature after you get used to it.

MEAL PREP FOR YOUR BUSY DAYS

Figuring out what to eat after a long shift can feel difficult and time-consuming. You're starving, your family is hungry, and everyone wants a meal on the table ASAP. You can avoid this headache by planning ahead and meal prepping dishes when you know you've got a busy day coming up. Meal prepping is simply the process of planning, cooking, and packaging your meals in advance. Here are just a few of the benefits of meal prepping:

- You'll save time and money.
- It's easier to manage your portions appropriately.
- You'll lower stress levels, develop a better relationship with food, and maybe even inspire others to do the same.
- It's a much more effective way to stay on track with your dietary or nutritional goals than throwing meals together at the last minute.

Meal prepping can seem like a daunting task, but here are some tips to help you make it work:

1. Start by making a plan for which meals you'll eat when.
2. Choose meals with overlapping ingredients to save you time and money. For example, you might pick two proteins—say, chicken breasts and ground beef—that you can use for multiple recipes in one week.

3. Keep your meal ideas simple. Save fancy meals for your days off or special celebrations. Use condiments and dressings to add different flavors when needed.
4. Make a grocery list based on your recipe choices and buy everything at once.
5. Try to cook multiple batches of a single recipe at once, instead of jumping from recipe to recipe.
6. If you can't actually cook a particular meal ahead of time, try to do as much prep as possible beforehand. For example, chopping your veggies the night before and storing in airtight containers will make your prep time the next evening much quicker.
7. Buy storage containers in various sizes. This will make it easy for you to store meals and snacks so you can grab and pack for your shifts.

This may seem like a lot of work, but you'll find the up-front planning is well worth the effort when you have dinner on the table in minutes!

TAKE THE STAIRS

Even though your body is likely busy most of your shift, you should also try to get regular exercise. That can be hard to fit into your daily schedule, though. Choosing to take the stairs at work, instead of the elevator or escalator, is a simple way to incorporate a few minutes of exercise on a daily basis. Those minutes accumulate over time and can significantly impact your physical health. If there are no stairs where you work, think about using stairs at other places you go, like a mall, hotel, or office building.

There are many mental and physical health benefits to taking the stairs. First, it can be a way to relieve stress before or during your shift. The release of endorphins can be a quick way to reduce built-up pressure and tension. Climbing stairs is considered a vigorous exercise, which means that it really gets your cardiovascular system pumping. Challenge yourself to take the stairs for one week and notice how adding this simple movement to your daily life can change the way you feel!

WEAR SUPPORTIVE SHOES

Being on your feet all day and practically running from task to task isn't the best thing for your body. You experience a lot of strain on your joints and muscle soreness from bending, carrying, and reaching. You can't change the job requirements, but you can change your shoes to be sure you've got a pair that is supportive, cushions your feet, and looks great too!

Everyone has different foot anatomy, gait, and stride. It's important to find the shoe that fits your foot properly. Many nurses wear sneakers, but some prefer clogs because they support the back and promote better posture. Others choose a variation of slides, like Crocs, because they're lighter and more breathable. Whatever you choose, make sure the shoe you wear is right for your body and job requirements. Find a shoe store near you that can analyze your gait and stride, as well as discuss your goals with the shoes. Marathon runners wouldn't run 26.2 miles in just any sneaker they find in their closet. They plan and take time to choose their running tools. The same should go for you! Proper footwear should be considered a part of your essential tool kit to optimize your work performance.

Wearing the right shoes at work will reduce the risk of plantar fasciitis, stress fractures, lower back pain, shin pain, and general muscle soreness. And comfortable, supportive shoes don't have to look dowdy—they can still be fashion-forward and geared to your style. Once you determine the type of shoe that works best for you, check out different brands, colors, and patterns so you can find something that matches your preferences and personality.

PRIORITIZE SLEEP

There's not one area of your mental, physical, and emotional health that isn't affected by your quality of sleep. The biggest challenge for nurses is that your world is so fast-paced that it can be difficult to unwind and fall asleep even when you're exhausted. Many nurses have conditioned their bodies to function while being chronically sleep-deprived.

Unfortunately, there are many detrimental effects of getting a low quality and quantity of sleep:

- Lower immunity
- Increased risk of diabetes, obesity, and depression
- Irritability
- Memory loss
- Lack of productivity

Most nurses don't realize that sleep deprivation is the origin of most of their health issues until it's too late. You deserve to rest and recharge, and your patients deserve a healthy, happy, and well-rested nurse! So how can you improve the situation? Here are some tips:

- Make a weekly plan on how you can schedule in enough hours of sleep (ideally six to eight hours).

- Go to bed at the right time to avoid getting a second wind.
- Expose yourself to more sunlight during the day to improve your natural circadian rhythm.
- If you work nights, invest in blackout shades and a comfortable eye mask so you can sleep during the day.
- Take a warm bath before bed to help loosen up tense muscles.
- Avoid screen time (yes, both TV and cell phone) for at least thirty minutes before bed.
- Have a strict caffeine curfew, preferably no less than six hours before bedtime.
- Drink caffeine-free tea, such as chamomile, before bed.
- Create a nice cool environment in your bedroom; using a fan or opening a window helps.
- Use a noise machine to block any sounds, especially if you need to sleep at a hospital.
- Turn on a diffuser with lavender essential oil to help you relax.
- Try meditating in bed to calm your inner chatter.

Your body, mind, and spirit will be grateful for any steps you take to improve the quality and quantity of your sleep!

REDUCE YOUR SUGAR INTAKE

Nurses often gravitate toward sugary foods and drinks because of their ability to boost energy levels quickly, but unfortunately, these energy boosts are followed by a speedy crash. This spike and crash of blood sugar levels is usually caused by refined sugars that are added to processed foods and drinks.

Refined sugars barely contain any nutritional value, plus they leave you less satiated and wanting to eat more. The peaks and valleys of sugar levels that refined sugars cause can also lead to fluctuations in mood, which can ultimately impact mental health. Along with mental health, your physical health is at risk. The spike in energy level that comes from sugar intake can be fleeting, leaving you fatigued and in a fog. Many medical conditions are also linked to excessive consumption of sugar, such as diabetes, obesity, and heart disease.

You probably know how to avoid obvious sources of sugar in your diet, like cake and ice cream, but it's important to be aware of hidden sugar in other foods. Here are some ways to reduce your refined sugar intake:

- Cut back on sugary beverages like sodas, energy drinks, sports drinks, fancy coffees, and juices.
- Choose low-sugar drink options like sparkling water with lemon, flavored seltzer water, unsweetened tea and coffee, fruit tea, and infused water with fruit.

- Avoid sugary-packed desserts. Try options like Greek yogurt topped with fruit, baked pear or apple with cinnamon, fruit salad, dark chocolate, or dates.
- Stay away from condiments and sauces with high sugar content, like ketchup. Instead use fresh or dried herbs, mustard, vinegar, fresh salsa, or pesto.
- Eat whole foods that haven't been processed or refined, and that are free of artificial sweeteners.
- Check for sugar in canned foods. Many canned foods use sugar as a preservative and for added flavor.
- Start your day with a low-sugar, high-fiber, and high-protein breakfast. Some ideas include oatmeal with nuts, cottage cheese topped with pineapple, eggs, avocado toast, or a fresh fruit salad.
- Eat more protein, fat, and fiber to help you stay satisfied and fuller for a longer period of time.
- Consider using natural sweeteners like honey and stevia.
- Don't go food shopping when you're hungry. This can lead to impulse purchases of sugary snacks and drinks.

As a nurse, you know that your body and brains need a certain amount of glucose to properly function. Natural sources of sugar, such as those from fruits, vegetables, grains, and dairy products, are what produce the steadiest amount of glucose to fuel you.

CREATE A HOME
WORKOUT ROUTINE

Exercise is such an important way to foster positive physical self-care. But finding the time with a nurse's schedule can be challenging. Not only do you have to consider the time it takes to complete the workout, but also the commute to and from the gym. Creating a home workout routine can cut out time and excuses!

At-home workouts may be intimidating at first, but when you find the routine that's right for you, it becomes a life-altering decision. You can schedule workouts on your days off, or even before or after a shift. Exercising at home can come in many forms: guided videos, premade programs, or a routine you build yourself.

Despite what many believe, workouts at home are just as effective without all the equipment you get from a gym. Depending on the exercises you're doing, simple equipment like a yoga mat, dumbbells, and resistance bands will suffice. Having equipment available allows you to mix it up between cardio and strength. You can even utilize items around the house as weights—try soup cans or gallons of water!

So where do you begin? Start by thinking about your physical health goals. Are you looking to lose weight, build muscle, or maintain overall health? Then decide how many times a week and when you will be exercising. Come up with a realistic time frame for your workouts; an hour might be a big stretch for you some days. After you've considered how you'll incorporate home workouts into your life, decide what kind of program would work best for you:

- **Try a guided workout.** Some people respond best to following a coach's instruction, so maybe a program with videos will be most effective. There are plenty of guided programs to choose from; look into memberships with companies like Beachbody, Sweat, Athlean-X, and Peloton.
- **See what's available on social media.** Many fitness social media accounts offer home workout programs that you can download and then do at your own speed. You can turn on your favorite jams and get to it whenever you like!
- **Create your own workout.** If guided options don't sound like your cup of tea, create your own. When building your own workout routine, focus on muscle groups like biceps, shoulders, legs, and so on. Incorporate high-intensity interval training (HIIT), cardio, weight lifting, dancing, stretching, and mobility as part of your daily routines to keep it fun!

The added bonus to home workouts is that you're in control of time, equipment, breaks, and level of toughness. Every day brings different circumstances, so having the freedom to adjust your workout can help you stick to your program regardless of the fluctuations in your life.

DON'T DRINK YOUR CALORIES

Even if you try to eat healthy foods, it can be easy to overlook the calories in your drinks. Sugary beverages like sodas, energy drinks, fancy coffees, and juices can have unexpectedly high calorie and sugar content. How often do you reach for one of these during your shift? These drinks are tasty and give you an instant mood and energy boost, but unfortunately, they aren't the best for your health.

Most people drink 500 to 600 calories per day, but those same calories can also equal a nutritious, filling, and brain-fueling lunch. When you choose to eat nutritious calories instead of drinking empty calories and sugar, you will feel more satisfied, energized, and prepared for your shift.

Your body is most efficient when you are properly hydrated. Here are some ways to help your fluid intake be healthier:

- Try switching one of your calorie-filled drinks for water.
- Instead of reaching for the fancy latte, try black coffee with almond milk and honey.
- Swap soda for seltzer water.
- If you need some added flair for your water, add some sliced fruit.

There are many easy alternatives to save calories and boost the nutritional value of your fluids; you just have to find what's best for you!

CHAPTER FOUR

Professional Self-Care

Nursing burnout is a common phenomenon in the healthcare community. Stress is something almost everyone deals with on a day-to-day basis, but chronic stress—like what you might experience as a nurse—can become burnout. Burnout often looks like overall physical, mental, and emotional exhaustion, followed by disengagement from your work or even your loved ones. Many nurses and nursing students experience burnout because of their high-intensity work environment and lack of work-life balance.

Unfortunately, burnout not only affects nurses—it also cascades onto the patients and the families they care for. Think of how a nurse's energy radiates as soon as they walk into a room—if that energy is low and frustrated, the whole vibe of the room changes. Understandably, there is a strong correlation between nursing burnout and an increased risk of illness and medical errors due to fatigue and distraction. Hospitals with high burnout rates also tend to have lower patient satisfaction overall.

The good news is that there are many ways to cope with and/or avoid burnout altogether. In this chapter, you will find topics on how to avoid professional burnout and build a supportive work environment, all while being a great nurse! Ideas like saying no to unwanted overtime, taking your lunch break, listening to a nursing podcast, and obtaining certifications that apply to your specialty can help keep you rested, engaged, and motivated. Encouraging and supporting your professional identity will help you take care of both yourself and your patients.

BRING SOME "HAPPY" TO YOUR WORKDAY

Whether you stay in one spot most of the day or are running all over a floor, your surroundings can impact your happiness and motivation. While you probably can't paint the walls, there are lots of other ways that you can make your professional world as positive and joyful as possible.

Bringing "happy" to the workspace may look different for everyone. Here are a few ideas to start with:

- Wear vibrantly colored compression socks.
- Bring in your favorite coffee for the break room.
- Carry a small piece of your favorite candy in your scrubs pocket.
- Hang a picture of your family, pet, or loved ones by your computer or on your locker.
- Invest in colorful pens and a new supply bag.
- Wear fun earrings or surgical scrub hats.
- Buy brightly colored sticky notes.
- Hang inspirational quotes in patient rooms.

No matter how you choose to infuse some joy into your day, you'll notice how the positive vibes spread to your patients and coworkers.

STAND UP FOR YOURSELF

Though most patients are considerate and grateful, once in a while you encounter someone in a bad mood. Think back on a time when you had a patient call you by an insulting name or yell at you for not getting something they wanted fast enough. Unfortunately, nurses deal with these kinds of confrontations regularly. If you don't create healthy boundaries with patients, it becomes easier to accept this bad behavior. Some nurses have difficulty finding balance between being assertive and reacting inappropriately. The ultimate goal is to stand up for yourself while still maintaining professionalism. Here's how to deal with two common scenarios:

- **Rude patients:** Read the patient and their situation. Are they being rude because they're frustrated or in a lot of pain? Try to be empathetic and understand why they're acting the way they are. It may be as simple as allowing them to voice their concerns, and having a clear conversation about expectations throughout their hospital stay. Most rude patients feel unheard, frustrated, and powerless.

- **Attention seekers:** If a patient is looking to escalate a situation in order to seek attention, then remaining levelheaded and emotionless may be the best approach. Calmly leave the room and be clear that you will return when they need help or are ready to behave more appropriately.

Constantly experiencing bad behavior from patients can lead to nursing burnout, so part of your professional self-care routine should include standing up for yourself. Set healthy boundaries with patients and assure them that your role is to help them, but not to put up with rudeness.

UPDATE YOUR RESUME YEARLY

Nursing is such a rewarding profession. But if working in your current practice, area of nursing, or location makes you feel empty or "stuck," it may be time to consider other options. Your current job does not have to be permanent. Don't be afraid to research other specialties, hospitals, or organizations. The beauty of nursing is that you have access to so many opportunities! You just have to discover what's right for you. However, the prospect of job-searching can feel overwhelming, especially if you haven't revised your resume for years.

Your resume needs to be kept fresh and up-to-date in order for you to feel confident entering the job market. Updating your resume yearly will ensure that it's always accurate if an opportunity were to arise. You advanced yourself professionally, and you should absolutely take all of the credit for it. Be proactive, and take an hour once a year to focus on revising your resume. As you review it, you can focus on these points:

- Review your job responsibilities and add to or update any new tasks you've taken on.
- Highlight recent awards or recognition.
- Update data points as necessary.
- Add new skills you've acquired and certifications you've received.

As you make these revisions, you may be able to remove or minimize jobs from farther back in your past to keep the document focused on your more recent experience.

Knowing that you have an updated resume ready to be sent gives you the freedom to explore any opportunity that comes knocking on your door.

LISTEN TO A NURSING PODCAST

Podcasts have become one of the most popular ways to learn new things and share experiences. The healthcare system is frequently changing, but nurses are so busy that it can be difficult to stay abreast of new information and techniques. Finding the time to read clinical nursing journals or a book that focuses on their specialty is challenging. Listening to a podcast is a great way to receive necessary information and content in an easy way. You can be doing dishes, driving to work, jogging, or taking a shower *and* enhancing your knowledge.

With hundreds of nursing podcasts to choose from, you are bound to find a few that resonate with you and your nursing goals. Some podcasts are based solely on professional knowledge and relaying high-quality information about a particular topic, while others are filled with fun and light nursing stories. The variety of categories covered by podcasts include nursing students' topics, NCLEX prep, healthy work culture, career enhancement, healthcare news, critical care nurse information, ER nurse topics, and so on.

Here are some of the top nursing podcasts to consider:

- **FreshRN.** This is a podcast founded by a nurse, covering topics such as nursing procedures, dealing with difficult patients and their families, personal experiences, and other tips on how to get through nursing.

- **Straight A Nursing.** This is a great resource for nurses and nursing students who want to enhance their knowledge.
- **Real Talk School of Nursing.** This podcast focuses on building a community of supportive nurses and nursing students based around shared experiences rather than content taught in school.
- **The Nurse Keith Show.** Here is one of the best podcasts for career management and development, personal growth, entrepreneurship, and multidisciplinary collaboration in nursing.
- **The Happy Traveler.** This podcast focuses on traveling nurses, health, family, education, and money.
- **EMCrit.** Hosted by an emergency room MD, this podcast discusses all things related to medical education on ER intensive care, trauma, and resuscitation.
- **The WoMed.** Short for "Women in Medicine," this podcast approaches nursing with humor and fun. It focuses on self-care, mental health, emerging healthcare trends, and education.
- **The Nursing Podcast (NRSNG).** This podcast helps nursing students prepare for the NCLEX.
- **Continulus Critical Care Nursing.** This podcast delivers the latest evidence-based practices by the leading experts in critical care nursing.

Once you find one (or more!) that interests you, make listening to it a part of your daily or weekly routine.

WRITE A THANK-YOU NOTE TO A COWORKER

Chances are, some weeks you're spending more time with your coworkers than your family. Your fellow nurses, ancillary staff, and patient care assistants all come together and form a big "work family." Yes, you have your individual patient assignments, but you depend on the help of others to get things done.

When a coworker goes above and beyond and lends you a hand when you need it the most, let them know they're appreciated. One way to show them how much their help meant to you is by composing a handwritten thank-you note. Depending on how significant the help was, you can purchase a card, or just write your thoughts on a cute sticky note and stick it on their computer.

This small, kind gesture goes a long way! Think about how you would feel if you received a handwritten note. It would motivate you to keep supporting your coworkers and might even make you more likely to ask for help when you need it. No nurse should drown during the shift, or skip a lunch break in order to finish their tasks. You can be the one who starts an inspiring trend of thank-you notes to improve the overall work environment.

SAY NO TO
UNWANTED OVERTIME

Overtime is a great way to make additional income to purchase something special or pay off a credit card bill. Taking on extra shifts when you want or need to is beneficial for you. But constantly accepting overtime because your unit is short-staffed and you feel obligated to can be a quick path to burnout. This situation might sound familiar: Your manager calls you on your day off because someone called in sick, begging you to come in and promising to give you a good assignment. You're put on the spot and probably make the decision to take the shift, even if you'd rather spend time with your family. You're thanked for being such a good team player at work...but your personal life is left behind.

It is important for your mental, physical, and emotional health to put yourself first and make an honest decision about working extra hours. Ask yourself: "Is this what I truly want?" If not, do not feel guilty about saying no. You can still be a great and loyal nurse and not accept every overtime shift you're offered.

Staying home when your body needs it will give you more time to reflect on your past shifts, think about ways you can improve your practice, and recharge so you can return to work at full capacity. Use the time to focus on your family, friends, self-care, or even to learn new information about your specialty. Taking the time you need away from work is an important part of professional self-care, so give yourself permission to enjoy it.

ASK FOR HELP

Let's say you arrive at work, review the list of tasks you need to accomplish throughout your shift...and realize that you already feel overwhelmed. Whether you work in a hospital, clinic, outpatient facility, operating room, or school, your duties can feel endless. That's why it's important to know when you can truly handle your workload on your own—and when the list is just *too* long and you need a helping hand.

Remember this: You are not alone. Nursing is a team effort. Asking for help is one of the most important skills you can learn as a nurse. It can feel difficult for many reasons: fear of looking incompetent, not knowing who to ask, feeling afraid of being judged, or worrying that you're a burden. But burnout can happen very quickly if you try to carry everything on your shoulders. You also need to put your patients' safety and well-being before your ego. If you don't know how to perform a skill or what a medication is used for, you'll need help to ensure patient safety.

Here are a few tips you can use to get the help you need and deserve:

- Know what responsibilities your nurse assistants have and what tasks can be delegated to them.
- Build positive relationships with ancillary staff. Everyone (from environmental workers to dietary staff to nurse assistants to administrative professionals) is an important part of the team.
- Create a mental note of which nurses you can go to for help on certain topics.
- Use your nursing education resources. Don't be afraid to call teachers or professors and ask any questions you may have, big or small.
- Make a list of tasks by priority. If you have more than two tasks that have to be done at the same time, ask a coworker to help you with the simplest one.

If you are drowning, speak up. Your coworkers are not mind readers. Don't expect them to start doing things without giving them direction. And most importantly, say "thank you" when someone helps you. Those two words go a long way.

BUILD GOOD RELATIONSHIPS WITH PHYSICIANS AND PROVIDERS

Nurses interact and communicate with multiple physicians and other providers on a daily basis. They discuss patient status, plan of care, and review orders. Unfortunately, not every conversation goes smoothly. Even though everyone has the patient's best interests in mind, parties may have different ideas about which approach is the right choice.

Nurses spend the most time with the patient, which makes you a great advocate for what you think is right. You have a good sense of how the patient responds to certain medications or interventions and how the patient has been progressing, and therefore are able to provide certain recommendations. Providers will most likely respond optimistically to your advice and be keener to put in orders you need if they have a good ongoing relationship with you. The building of trust and rapport takes time, but it's worth the effort both for patient care and your own success and happiness at work.

There are a few ways you can start building a friendly relationship with your patient's providers. Here are some easy-to-implement ideas:

- When they walk into a patient room, introduce yourself by stating your name and title.
- If you're not sure who they are, ask for their name and what service they work for. It's always good to know what specialties are attending to your patient.
- If you have anything to contribute about the patient or their care, volunteer it respectfully.
- After their visit, take some time to discuss the patient's plan of care and what recommendations you have, if any.

Don't be afraid to speak up; you are all on the same team! The more times you engage with physicians and providers, the more you will both develop trust for each other. A better rapport will lead to better communication and improved patient outcomes.

PRACTICE YOUR INTERVIEWING SKILLS

It is easy to stay at a job for years, even if you're unhappy. People get comfortable with what they know, and venturing out to the unknown can feel intimidating. One way to feel more comfortable with searching for a new job is knowing that your interviewing skills are sharp. (You should also update your resume—see the Update Your Resume Yearly entry in this chapter for more information on that topic.)

Employers are constantly changing what they look for in an ideal candidate, so the questions they ask are different than they were years ago. Nursing interviews often incorporate clinical scenario questions, and we're all aware of how often evidence-based practice changes in medicine. Staying abreast of the latest medical information and interviewing strategies will make you feel more at ease when the time comes to look for a new job.

There are many ways to practice your interviewing skills without the help of a professional or coach. Here are a few examples:

- If you have a company or job in mind, research them and their mission statement ahead of your interview. It is always important to show the interviewer that you did your homework—it will prove how invested you are.

- Look up common general interview questions and brainstorm your responses. You don't have to memorize something word for word, but be sure you know how you'll handle the major topics that often arise.
- Come up with questions you would ask the interviewer about the company—possibly regarding benefits, hours, work culture, sick time, or salary.
- Think about your potential answers to clinical questions they may ask regarding your specific unit. For example, if you're interviewing for a position on a cardiac unit, practice clinical situations involving complications with cardiac patients and how you would intervene.
- Practice your posture and body language. (These skills are important to run through with someone else.) First impressions are invaluable, and how you communicate verbally and nonverbally is important. Aim for a firm handshake, sit up straight, lean forward slightly to indicate interest, avoid crossing your legs or arms, suppress fidgeting, and maintain good eye contact.
- When you're ready, rehearse a mock interview with a friend or partner. Rehearsing will lessen your interview-day jitters and allow you to get someone else's feedback on your answers.

These preparation tips for interviews will give you the confidence to apply for any nursing job you want!

LIST YOUR CAREER GOALS

Just as in any other career, it's important to have both long- and short-term goals. Long-term goals help shape the arc of your career, while short-term goals are the steps that help you move along your path. Maybe your goal is continuing education, getting a higher salary, or obtaining a new certification. Creating a plan for how to reach those goals will allow you to play an active role in your future.

Grab a pen and start writing. First make a list of a few long-term goals and a realistic date when you expect to achieve them. Now focus on one goal at a time and think of smaller steps that can help you move closer to that finish line.

Think of short-term goals as stepping-stones to bigger ones. For example, if your long-term goal is to become a family nurse practitioner, you might first check out master's programs in your area (assuming you are already an RN), choose one and enroll in it, select classes for your first term, and so on. These short-term goals will make your long-term goals seem more attainable, and provide you with a timeline and the opportunity to celebrate your success with rewards throughout the process. These interim achievements will help you stay motivated despite any obstacles thrown your way.

Once you begin working toward a goal, you'll find yourself having more direction and purpose. And once you achieve one goal, you'll be that much more motivated and confident to go after the next one.

TAKE YOUR LUNCH BREAK

In a traditional desk job, a break is scheduled and becomes a part of the daily routine. In nursing, sometimes "taking a break" only happens by luck or chance! You probably start the shift with good intentions to sit and eat something healthy, but then get consumed in patient care, multidisciplinary rounds, admissions, and discharges. Your duties are endless and you can accidentally work the entire shift without a break.

One reason it's challenging to schedule in breaks is the unpredictability of the job. Anything can happen on the spur of the moment and some tasks truly are life-or-death. Patient safety and health is priority, but you also have to know when to put yourself first. Not taking your break can lead to fatigue, burnout, mental fog, medication errors, and unhappiness. When a nurse is not at their best, patient safety and satisfaction are at risk! The old cliché "you can't pour from an empty cup" should be the slogan for nursing. If the day really is super busy, work with a colleague to cover you while you eat, then return the favor.

Taking your full lunch break at once may not be realistic some days, so make a plan to take multiple short breaks if that is more attainable. Taking a break should be a concrete part of your shift, but it's up to you to prioritize it and hold it as a standard.

OBTAIN EXTRA
CERTIFICATIONS OR DEGREES

Your registered nurse license permits you to provide care for patients, but is the minimum requirement for professional nurses. Earning additional certifications or degrees that apply to your specialty is a way for you to advance your nursing career without going back to school full-time. Adding the extra letters to your name is rewarding, and also sets you apart from other nurses. This especially applies when you're interviewing for a new position.

Passing the NCLEX is something to be proud of, but passing certification exams feels different! It validates you as a nurse and gives you the confidence and deeper knowledge you need to stand out at work. Obtaining certifications also keeps you abreast of the latest evidence-based practices and gives you the opportunity to practice at a higher level. These certifications will give you more of an understanding about symptom management, interventions, complications, and treatment plans specific to your patient population. Some examples of additional certifications or degrees you might consider include Bachelor of Science in Nursing (BSN), Nurse Practitioner (Family, Adult Gerontology, Acute, Neonatal, Psychiatric), Nurse Anesthetist (CRNA), Certified Nurse-Midwife (CNM), Clinical Nurse Specialist (CNS), Nurse Educator, or Nurse Executive, or programs in Healthcare Policy, Nursing Leadership and Management, Population Health, and Nursing Informatics.

Being able to claim yourself as a certified nurse proves your commitment to professional advancement in the nursing field. Some organizations even offer incentive compensation to get certified—so ask your manager or human resources department about that! Do a little research on what is offered for your specialty and get to work.

KEEP AN OPEN DIALOGUE
WITH YOUR MANAGER

Having issues on your unit or within your nursing department isn't a rare occurrence. Coworkers have disagreements, mistakes are made, doctors can become aggressive about patient care, and you may simply be overworked. Or, the question on your mind might be related to your career path or new opportunities on the horizon. Instead of letting these things fester, make your manager aware to see what solutions are possible.

Here are a few tips that can yield positive results and resolution in your interactions with your boss:

- Managers don't like surprises, so when you have an issue you want to discuss, alert them and try to set a time and date to talk instead of barging into their office unannounced. Find a mutually agreeable time, hopefully when neither one of you is busy putting out other fires on the unit. Try to be aware of what else they are dealing with in order to set up the best possible conversation.
- Going to a manager early on is the best approach. It wouldn't be fair to expect a resolution when a problem has already escalated too far.
- Have a clear plan of what you are going to say and how you will state your case. There shouldn't be any irrelevant information shared or beating around the bush.

- Body language is very important. Sit up tall in your chair, restrain from fidgety movements, and keep good eye contact.
- Outline the issue as objectively as possible, and be sure to mention what you have already done to try to resolve it on your own. If you made a mistake, be honest and own up to it.
- If the issue is a conflict with a coworker, be prepared to have a conversation with the other person in order to reach the best resolution. Open communication is always key in the nursing profession. Nurses depend on each other to work as an effective team, and unresolved conflict can be a slippery slope to poor patient outcomes. After you get advice and guidance from your manager, you can proceed to this step.
- In order to get used to talking to your manager, you might want to set up a periodic check-in meeting so you don't let things build up. Whether it's once a month or once a quarter, setting up a time to talk can be beneficial for both of you.

The key takeaway is to approach your manager early, with confidence and integrity. Keeping this open dialogue will help them help you with any issue, big or small.

LEARN HOW TO RESOLVE CONFLICT WITH A COWORKER

Conflict between coworkers is inevitable in the nursing world. With a melting pot of personalities, attitudes, and stressful situations, something is bound to get misinterpreted, and that's where conflict arises. Unresolved conflict is one of the biggest hindrances to productivity and workplace satisfaction.

Unfortunately, people in all industries aren't often taught how to address conflict, so instead they choose to avoid it, gossip behind each other's backs, or just give the other person the cold shoulder. This solution isn't healthy, and in nursing can lead to poor patient outcomes. Nurses rely on each other to get through the shift, and having unresolved conflict can impede workflow. Picture an emergency situation with one of your patients, where you are calling for help and the nurse you had an argument with yesterday is the only one available. That nurse will likely still come and help, of course, but will you share optimal communication and teamwork? Chances are it will be an awkward interaction that can ultimately impact patient care.

The next time you are in conflict with a coworker, try to calm down first, then try these resolution tips:

- Speak face-to-face when addressing the issue. Conversations through text, email, or other people can easily get misinterpreted and end in worse conflict.

- Don't talk about the situation with other coworkers. The most destructive way to hinder resolving conflict in a healthy way is having the other person hear that you were spreading the story to others.
- Suggest a meeting spot where you will both feel comfortable speaking. It should be a private area where both of you can share thoughts freely.
- Listen and empathize as you talk. There are multiple sides to a story, and that person might have something going on behind the scenes that you were totally unaware of. Actively listen to what the other person has to say and read nonverbal cues. It's important to make sure you truly hear other people's feelings and perspective.
- Don't let your ego get in the way. Have an open mind to alternative solutions.
- It's okay to agree to disagree. You may not understand each other's views, and that's okay too. Concluding this way is a form of resolution as long as you're both on the same page—but if the same situation is bound to come up again, try a little harder to find a resolution you can both live with.
- Know when to involve a manager. If the situation gets out of hand and you are unable to come to a resolution on your own, seek additional help. Sometimes all you need is guidance and an unbiased point of view to help you both see a way forward.

Conflict is uncomfortable and unpleasant, but working through it is far better than ignoring it or making it worse. The more practice you have at finding resolutions, the less intimidated you will feel when conflicts arise.

SCHEDULE IN STUDY BREAKS

Being a nursing student is incredibly challenging. Even if you are already a nurse and are studying to become a nurse practitioner, educator, or nurse anesthetist, entering a different realm of nursing can be overwhelming. Long study sessions and sleepless nights may seem par for the course, but they can also be toxic to your body over a long period of time.

Breaks are crucial to effective study sessions for several reasons:

- Taking a moment to walk away gives your brain time to recover and refresh, boosting your mood and energy.
- Studying for hours on end can lead to extreme fatigue that decreases productivity over time.
- Doing something fun or active during your breaks can give you the energy you need to continue your sessions strong.

Here are a few short activities that can recharge your batteries while studying:

- Take a five-minute walk outdoors.
- Eat a brain-fueling snack.
- Take fifteen minutes to call a friend.
- Grab a cup of coffee or another beverage.
- Listen to your favorite song.

Hitting the books is admirable, but taking short breaks will actually help you retain more information over the long run.

JOIN A STUDY GROUP

Joining or creating a study group can be one of the most beneficial and rewarding things you do during your time in nursing school. Having the ability to discuss difficult topics with your classmates can help you grasp the information and be better prepared for your exams. Being able to teach the concepts you do understand to others can also make you feel confident when you need it the most!

In order to have the most success with a study group, you need to gather the right people. Find classmates who have similar learning methods and academic goals. Here are some tips for creating a diligent study group:

- Start early in the semester. Try spending the first week or two of class making new friends and getting them interested in studying together. Pay attention to who participates in class and who has done the required reading beforehand.
- Once you have an idea of who you may want to include, gather their contact information at the end of class. Determine which days are best to meet and plan to meet on a regular basis—once or twice a week.
- Starting a group chat via text messaging or email is an effective way to remind people of study meetups and keep people accountable, and also serves as a platform to share study resources.

Being a part of a study group will encourage you and give your grades a boost—and you'll make friends along the way!

START AN EMPLOYEE-OF-THE-MONTH PROGRAM

Nurses work tirelessly to provide optimal care for their patients. You go above and beyond, prioritizing their safety and progress. Regardless of how much you do for your patients and for your unit, you may not get the recognition you deserve. It is important to foster a work environment that promotes incentive and high performance levels. Starting an Employee-of-the-Month (EOM) program for the staff (including ancillary staff and providers, if applicable) can shift the work culture significantly.

A common reason for nurses to leave their job is feeling overworked and underappreciated, but an EOM program can help address that feeling. Plus, staff will be more inclined to help each other, improve unit morale, maintain a positive attitude, and provide better patient care. Monthly recognition identifies diligence and hard work, motivating other employees to do the same. This plan generally works best at larger offices, but you can also adapt it for smaller groups, perhaps by changing the frequency of the awards.

There are a few things to take into consideration to assure a fun and effective EOM program that will be sustainable:

- Bring up the idea of an EOM program to your manager and/or human resources liaison. Before you approach them, come up with a plan of action. Together you can establish goals and desired outcomes for the program—like improved employee satisfaction.

- Set up rules and expectations. The EOM is supposed to be the model employee for the rest of the workforce. Make a list of what the ideal EOM looks like for your unit. If you choose staff members randomly each month, the program will quickly lose credibility.
- Decide on a system for voting. You can have a ballot box in the break room, create a special EOM email, or submit a nomination form in a box on your manager's door.
- Decide on a reward for the winner of the month. The reward can be small, like candy, a gift card for coffee, or a badge reel pin.
- If possible, set up an EOM recognition wall or picture frame where you can announce and publicize the winner. This will keep the staff well engaged and generate even greater interest!

An important part of this program is its promotion. Once you create the program, it's vital that you inform the staff of the entire process—from the qualifications needed to receive the award to how the winner will get chosen. Getting the appreciation you deserve feels amazing! When done correctly, an EOM program can provide positive outcomes and reduce staff burnout.

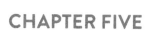

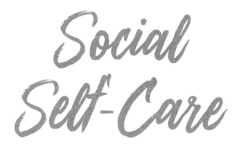

CHAPTER FIVE

Self-care doesn't always have to be a solo act. Social self-care— in other words, spending time with the people you love—is also a vital way to recharge. Despite nurses' busy schedules, days off do come, so be sure you see loved ones on some of those days.

After all, you're not only a nurse, of course. Mom, dad, son, daughter, sister, brother, cousin, friend, coach, volunteer, activist, athlete, community leader—whatever your many titles may be, they're all equally important in your life. Social self-care involves activities that nurture and deepen those relationships and roles. Whether you plan a dinner party with your family, host a game night with neighbors, visit a relative you haven't seen in a while, or sign up for a 5K race supporting a worthwhile cause, you'll be interacting with others in a fun way. Most of the ideas in this chapter don't require loads of time or money—just use your creativity and make the most of the resources you have available to you.

Connecting with others fosters feelings of love, gratitude, acceptance, and compassion, which are all necessary components of being an awesome nurse! This is why it's so important to use your days off as opportunities to practice social self-care, and recharge yourself.

GO BOWLING
WITH COWORKERS

Bowling can be a fun team-building activity, and also a great way to develop or deepen relationships among coworkers. Whereas you get to know your colleagues at work through common ground—long shifts and challenging patients—interacting in a low-stress, fun environment is a totally different experience. An activity like this will benefit your personal friendships, and also help build a more trusting professional relationship.

Don't know where to begin? Pick a date and time that is convenient and a location that is near work. Leaving a sign-up sheet in the break room is a simple way to engage coworkers and an easy way to make everyone aware of the event. You can also create an electronic invitation that can be sent via text or work email. Call the bowling alley in advance and figure out logistics regarding pricing, food, and drinks.

A night out of bowling reinforces teamwork and will bring you and your nurse friends even closer. Whether you take it seriously (matching shirts, anyone?) or make it as silly as possible (give an award for the lowest score), getting to know your colleagues outside of work is a great way to see and enjoy them as full people, not just nurses.

HOST A NEIGHBORHOOD FOOD DRIVE

Hunger is an issue that can be happening right under your nose, in your own neighborhood. You probably even witness food insecurity in your patients. Nurses are such a giving group of people, so why not take those qualities and apply them outside of the workplace as well? Hosting a food drive in your neighborhood will allow you to give back, while also strengthening your relationships with and connection to the people in your community.

Whether you want to host a traditional drive with nonperishable foods, or a virtual collection of funds for your local food bank, you can make a huge difference in your community. Collecting supplies and funds helps food pantries and soup kitchens in your area keep their shelves stocked to feed those in need. A local food drive can also raise awareness about hunger in your neighborhood, and motivate others to help.

Organizing a food drive is simple, and you can host it on your own or collaborate with friends and family. Here's what to do:

1. Contact your local food bank. Every location works differently, so getting specific details on what they need and how you can support them is the best way to start. They may also be able to provide you with useful advice for hosting the best food drive.
2. Select a date to begin and end your drive; it can be as short as a few hours or as long as a month.

3. Decide what you're collecting. For a virtual fundraiser, monetary donations would be the only form of contribution. But for a traditional drive, you can request popular items like canned, boxed, or bagged nonperishable food items.
4. Decide where the drop-off location will be. You can use your front porch or maybe ask a local business if you can use their parking lot during hours when they're closed.
5. You may need volunteers to stay at the collection site at certain times, so make sure to plan accordingly.
6. Get people engaged and aware of the food drive by creating flyers and posting them around the neighborhood. You may also want to contact your local newspaper for more publicity. Spread your announcement at least two weeks in advance to give people time to schedule in time for their support.
7. Decide how you'll get the donations to the food bank. If you've collected money, it might already go right to the organization itself. For food donations, sometimes the organization will pick up boxes of donations for you; others will want you to deliver it to their location.

This social self-care activity is rewarding and beneficial for you *and* your community. You can feel good about making a difference in someone's life by just providing daily necessities.

RESOLVE A FEUD

Relationships—whether with family, friends, coworkers, or your partner—take effort. No bond is perfect, and there will always be misunderstandings and disagreements along the way. Learning how to deal with conflict is a worthwhile endeavor, in both your personal and professional lives. (For tips on resolving conflict at work, see the Learn How to Resolve Conflict with a Coworker entry in Chapter 4.) Fostering good communication with a loved one, especially about difficult situations, will make you both feel more fulfilled and stronger in the relationship.

Before calling up your friend in a rage because he forgot your birthday, take a second to step back and think about how to successfully resolve the issue. Here are some tips for moving through a conflict in a productive way:

- Talk *and* listen. Effective communication involves accurately relaying information to the other person, but also actively listening to what they have to say. Remember to consider their feelings and perspective, because everyone has a right to how they feel.
- Be clear and precise when it's your turn to speak. Don't beat around the bush when trying to get something across, as this only confuses the other person.
- If you're having this conversation in person, be aware of your nonverbal cues—body language speaks louder than words.
- Try your best to remain calm and levelheaded throughout the conversation.

Coming to a resolution might take time and compromise, but it will be well worth it. Deepening relationships is a key part of social self-care, and having unresolved feuds with others is not beneficial for anyone.

VOLUNTEER FOR
A LOCAL CHARITY

Free time doesn't have to always mean *you* time. A big part of social self-care is spending time developing relationships and helping others within your community. Volunteering your time for a local organization can foster meaningful relationships with people who you otherwise may never meet. Choose an organization that aligns with your interests and values and see what type of help they need.

The complexities of nursing may leave you depleted on your days off. But volunteering and serving others in need can actually energize you! This act is rewarding in itself—and can also help you recharge your batteries for shifts to come. Whether you choose an animal shelter, food bank, environmental charity, or something else, you will feel like part of the solution in helping your community.

Call the organization you'd like to help ahead of time and sort out a volunteering option that suits you and your schedule. Tell a few friends or coworkers and see if they would like to join! Involving loved ones will also give you something special to bond over. You can make such a huge difference by volunteering, and that experience is empowering and humbling all at once.

GO ON A DATE NIGHT WITH YOUR PARTNER

It's easy to come home from a shift exhausted and disengaged—not exactly the best mindset to connect with your partner. So, how can you elevate your relationship with your partner and nurture this aspect of your social self-care? Go on a date night!

Plan to have a full evening to yourselves, with zero interruptions. Date night doesn't have to be pricey or fancy. You can stay in, cook dinner together, and watch a movie. Or, plan an adventurous night with a fun new activity that you can bond over. Let go of any excuses you have running through your mind like lack of time, the hassle of finding a babysitter, or being too tired. Speak to your partner and plan a date night in advance, so you can both make it work and look forward to it.

Scheduling in the time to spend meaningful time with your partner is key to a healthy relationship. Focus on simply enjoying each other's company, good conversation, laughs, and intimacy. If you can, make date night into a monthly ritual! It's important to step away from nursing and enhance the relationship between you and your support person.

ESTABLISH HEALTHY BOUNDARIES

Boundaries might seem like an afterthought when you're a nurse, since you may be very intimately involved with your patients' bodily functions. But every type of boundary—physical, emotional, and verbal—is still important to define and maintain.

Establishing personal boundaries within your relationships increases your self-esteem, reduces stress and anxiety, and fosters better communication. On the other hand, in the absence of proper boundaries, others will behave however they think is appropriate. Think about a time when your manager asked you to take an extra shift that you wanted to decline, but you said yes anyways. Or maybe there was a time when a doctor was disrespectful and you didn't stand up for yourself. Personal boundaries need to be set in order to avoid situations like these.

So what are boundaries and how do you create them for yourself? Defining boundaries is a way for you to determine what you will and will not accept from others. There are several types of boundaries:

- **Physical boundaries** include things like personal space, your body, and privacy. If someone is standing too close or touches you inappropriately, verbalize your discomfort and establish a boundary between you and that person.

- **Emotional boundaries** involve disassociating your feelings from someone else's. A few violations include letting other people tell you what you "should be" feeling, sacrificing your own needs to satisfy someone else, and blaming others for your problems.
- **Verbal boundaries** refer to how someone speaks to you. For example, if profanities or certain comments make you feel uncomfortable, you should say so. You have the right to make your own choices about how others talk to you. Setting strong verbal boundaries for yourself will protect your integrity and self-esteem.

Most people, especially nurses, have a difficult time with creating healthy boundaries, so be gentle with yourself if it doesn't feel comfortable at first. It might help you to frequently remind yourself that you are worthy of your own identity, thoughts, and values. If you are worried that standing up for your boundaries might disrupt a relationship, try not to let that hold you back. Chances are, your interactions with that person already make you feel resentful, anxious, stressed, or guilty—and those are signs that you need to make a change anyway. Steps to build better boundaries are rooted from understanding what your own limits are. You are worthy of happiness and are in control of your behaviors and feelings.

Once you define what healthy boundaries work the best for you, the interactions you have with people at work and in your personal life will begin to shift. This shift may be unpleasant at first, but in the long run, it will lead to a healthier social environment for you.

VISIT A RELATIVE

It's essential to foster good relationships with the people who mean the most to you, whether that's your favorite cousin or a beloved great-aunt. Relatives have so much to teach you, including family traditions and old stories. Maintaining a close bond doesn't have to mean calling them on a daily basis to catch up. It can simply be taking a few hours of your day once in a while to chat over coffee.

As a nurse, you know how important it is to live life to the fullest. Each day is a gift to be cherished and should not be taken for granted. We have the privilege of witnessing the cycle of life—birth and death—on a weekly basis. The opportunity to visit a family member may not always be there. During your time together, you can reminisce on beautiful life memories; this alone can leave you with a joyful feeling. But you can also make new memories to hold with you forever. You'd be surprised at what sitting at a table, talking, can do for your emotional and social well-being. Time spent building family relationships is never time wasted. So schedule in the time, and do it while you can!

DO A WINE TASTING

A glass of your favorite wine can take the edge off a tough shift and set the mood for a relaxing evening. While enjoying a glass of wine alone is satisfying, sharing it with friends is even better! Doing a wine tasting with friends is a great way to promote social self-care. If you're not able to meet in person, you can even do a virtual wine tasting from the comfort of your own home.

To plan a wine tasting, research wineries near you that host tastings or that will supply a "wine kit" that can be delivered to various homes if you're doing it virtually. Select the list of wines you'll taste, and look up a few facts about each one so you'll know what to expect. To make it into a more interactive event, give each guest a wine to research and lead the discussion on—this can be really fun if everyone is willing to participate. Keep things casual and easygoing, so you can let go of the day's stress with a few glasses of wine and a good time with friends.

PLAN A DINNER PARTY

Planning a dinner party is a fun way to spend quality time with your friends and family. It's all too easy to let days and weeks go by without spending meaningful time with family, and that can put a strain on your well-being. A key part of social self-care is strengthening relationships with others around us, and what better way than to share delicious food, drinks, and laughs with the ones you love?

Hosting a dinner party may seem intimidating, but it doesn't need to be! Here are a few tips that can guide you to a smooth evening:

1. **Pick a date.** Having a set date will give you and your guests time to prepare. It may be a good idea to choose a date far in advance to give your family and friends enough time to clear their schedules.
2. **Decide who to invite.** When making a guest list, try to invite people who will get along well and have a great time together, including you.

3. Choose a theme! Themes are a fun way to create a cohesive menu, online invitations, decor, and cocktails. Your guests will be sure to get excited over it. Consider preparing make-ahead recipes so you are not doing a lot of active cooking while your guests are there. That way, you can relax and have fun too!
4. Write out a shopping list based on the menu you came up with and go to the store. Don't forget any accessories or paper goods you might need.
5. Prepare your home with a welcoming ambiance. Apart from the decor, consider adding a few candles, low lighting, pleasant background music, and comfortable seating.
6. Relax and enjoy yourself and your guests!

A dinner party is a fun (and delicious) way to relax and enjoy time away from work.

REACH OUT TO A COWORKER WHO HAD A BAD SHIFT

All nurses have a bad shift every once in a while. After a bad shift, you might go home and replay everything that happened, wondering what you could have done differently. You probably question your strengths as a nurse, which may have nothing to do with why the shift went so poorly. Just as in your nonwork life, it's natural to have good and bad days, but it's how you cope with them that makes all the difference.

After a bad shift, don't you feel better when you talk to someone who understands what you went through, like a fellow nurse friend? One way to practice social self-care is by being a listening ear to a coworker who needs to vent. Releasing all of the emotions that arise from a bad shift can be so helpful to a stressed nurse. Your coworker may just need to unload everything they're feeling to someone who's been there before. Being there for a work friend can really change that person's day and also strengthen your relationship. Providing comfort for others will also open doors for others to help you someday when you really need it.

CALL SOMEONE WHO HAS BEEN ON YOUR MIND

Because of your overly packed schedule with work, errands, and activities, a quick text message might be the fundamental go-to for communication. While keeping up with relationships through texts is valuable, there is nothing like an old-fashioned phone call. Whether you're thinking about an old friend, sibling, or other family member, a conversation over the phone may bring you that connection you've been craving. Without this "old school" way of communication, you lose a special emotional connection that is key in social relationships.

A phone conversation can be minutes or hours long; it's really up to you. Some people find it to be an annoyance when the phone rings, and may not even pick up, so try scheduling the call so you both have carved out time to catch up. If you have a long commute home, use the time to your advantage!

Speaking to someone over the phone can easily be made into a routine—especially if you build it into your daily activities. Invest in wireless headphones to make it easier for you to cook, clean, do laundry, or go for a walk while on the phone. Nurses are great at multitasking, so use those skills to your advantage here! Maintaining good relationships takes effort, but something as simple as a phone call can make it less complicated.

EVALUATE WHO YOU SURROUND YOURSELF WITH

Who you surround yourself with matters. It's no secret that you are influenced by others; it's part of human nature. Relationships are essential for feelings of acceptance and comfort, but also to help guide you through life. Still, how often have you stepped back and evaluated who's around you? We often overlook the impact our connections with others have on every aspect of our lives. These connections can work in both ways—good and bad. For example, you are more likely to think negatively about your workplace if your immediate coworkers only have negative things to say. On the other hand, if you're intimidated by applying to school to advance your career, but your friend has done it and is constantly inspiring you to be better, you may be more inclined to go for it!

Taking a closer look at your network can help you better understand yourself and your behaviors. If your network of people demonstrates specific behaviors, that can change your perception of what normal behavior is, and eventually you mold your behaviors accordingly. Who you surround yourself with should push you to elevate your life. You should strive to make each other better personally, professionally, financially, and spiritually. Think about a time when you were treated unfairly at work and the shift made you question the nursing profession. Who did you vent to and how did it end? If you went to someone who is a positive influence in your life, chances are it ended with you feeling much better.

Consider the normal attitudes, feelings, and behaviors of the people you spend most of your time with. Challenge yourself by writing down your preferred behaviors, and assess if they are in alignment. Take a few minutes to ask yourself a few questions about the people around you:

- Are they motivating you?
- Would you consider them to be positive influences?
- Do they help you feel stronger when you're feeling down?
- Do they occasionally push you out of your comfort zone?
- Are they inspiring you to be your best self?
- Do they share common goals with you?

When evaluating who you surround yourself with, don't be afraid of being selective. It may be challenging to make decisions about who you need to disconnect from, but it'll be worth it for your own self-care. Friendship groups are powerful. Be sure you are spending time with people you admire rather than those who bring you down. You deserve to be the best *you* there is, and negative relationships will never get you there.

GO ON A HIKE WITH FRIENDS

Going on a hike is a beautiful experience to share with friends, and is also beneficial for your physical health. You will all make memories that can last a lifetime and can witness some amazingly beautiful spots out in nature.

If you've never hiked before, it may seem intimidating, but there's nothing to be nervous about. Whether you think you're not in shape or are scared of getting lost, you can plan a hike that matches everyone's ability level. This is meant to be a low- to moderate-impact exercise, focused on enjoying the company of friends. Do some research on the intensity and length of the hike before you go. Before the big day, pack a comfortable backpack with the essentials, such as adequate water, healthy snacks, a small first aid kit, insect repellent, a hat, sunblock, and hand sanitizer.

If you have space, pack an extra clothing layer just in case the weather changes. Wearing the right shoes can have a significant impact on your experience. You want to avoid sore feet and blisters as much as possible. Also, make sure your shoes have enough traction to prevent slipping throughout the hike. Wear tall socks for extra protection, and opt for lighter-colored clothing to help detect ticks or other dangerous bugs.

Take your time finishing the hike; this is not a race. Enjoy the beautiful scenery along the journey, and maybe even set up a picnic when you reach a lovely spot. Plan for this day to be fun and relaxing; don't put any pressure on yourself or your friends to perform a certain way. Instead, focus on reconnecting with your friends and sharing a few laughs along the way.

TAKE A FRIEND
OUT FOR COFFEE

Sometimes the best ways to develop or maintain a friendship is over a simple in-person conversation. Sure, text messages and emails are convenient, but socializing in person is so much better. Body language, laughter, and physical touch truly help form a stronger bond. Meeting up with a friend and treating them to a caffeine boost is fun and can lift both of your moods. You can both use this time to vent about life's woes, laugh about a funny story, or maybe even gain a new perspective on issues you've been struggling with. Taking an old friend out for coffee is great, but you can also use this activity to make new friends!

Be open as you chat, and try to get to know each other on a new level. Social self-care doesn't have to be complicated, expensive, or time-consuming—something as simple as a conversation over a cup of coffee can change your outlook on your whole week.

HOST A GAME NIGHT

Nurses spend most of their time being serious, diligent, and vigilant people at work. Tasks like dosing medication, stabilizing patients, dealing with family members, and managing admissions and discharges leave very little time for fun and games. You deserve to let loose and enjoy a fun-filled game night every once in a while! A game night is a great way to interact with a group of loved ones all at once. The friendly competition adds an energetic vibe that will surely have everyone cheerful and laughing.

Before you send out a group invitation text or email, there are a few things to take into consideration:

- Invite a big group, preferably an even number of people, so you can make teams more easily. Make sure that the group of people invited are enthusiastic about a game night and are willing to participate.
- The last thing you want is a buzz kill an hour into the night, with everyone arguing over what games to play, so choose the game(s) in advance, and make the guests a part of the process. For example, you can provide options and have everyone choose their top three games via an online poll.

- Don't start the games right away; instead, start the night off with socializing, getting everyone their favorite drinks, and catching up. This will lighten the mood and get the guests comfortable with each other before you dive into competition.
- Serve finger foods that don't require anyone to sit down with a plate. You don't need to serve a full dinner—think chips or veggies and dip, cheese and crackers, premade appetizers, and cut-up fruit. And don't forget a variety of beverages for your guests to choose from.
- Make sure you have enough comfortable seating, and an area where you will play the game(s).

There's nothing like spending quality time laughing with people you love. A raucous game night can be just the ticket to forgetting all about work worries.

WRITE AN APPRECIATION LETTER TO YOUR PARTNER

Nurses spend a lot of time at work, away from their partners. Plus, since you're not working a traditional desk job, there is little time during workdays to share emotions. Even your days off may be filled with chores and errands, and they might not sync up with your partner's days off. Sweet text messages and short notes around the house are thoughtful ways to show appreciation, but sometimes you need to say a little more.

Think about the last time your partner did something meaningful and special for you. How did that make you feel? Most likely, happy and loved! Writing down these feelings in a letter to your partner can deepen your relationship, which is a positive form of social self-care for both of you.

Getting into the right mental space is very important to be able to share the most accurate feelings. Set the mood with a few candles, light music, and a comfortable seat. Maybe go through a few of your favorite pictures and reminisce on beautiful memories you've shared together. If you've recently overcome a challenge in your relationship, focus on how thankful you are for their support and dedication. Or, if you simply just want to touch on a few of their best qualities, consider making a list beforehand to organize the letter a little better. You can also have a theme to your letter—for example, "thank you for everything you do for me," "thank you for supporting me during a tough time," "thank you for being you," or "thank you for listening to me when I need to vent." You can buy a card from a store, type it up on your laptop, or handwrite it on special paper.

Really try to make your letter extra thoughtful and kind. Nurses have very challenging days and nights, and having a partner to lean on is something special and should be cherished. Your partner will really like getting acknowledged and being shown how much they're appreciated. This activity will leave you and your partner stronger and more connected!

PLAN A ROAD TRIP

Is work making you stressed and overwhelmed? A road trip is such a fun and refreshing way to strengthen relationships with friends, family, or your partner. It allows time away from the "real world" and responsibilities, giving you the opportunity to bond uninterruptedly. Windows down, sightseeing, singing along to your favorite music, and enjoying snacks along the way—it sounds magical! Let's start planning:

- Decide who will be your traveling partners on this trip, and agree on the dates and length of time.
- Consider the type of road trip you want to experience. Think of sticking to a certain theme to make it easier for planning: popular tourist road trips, national parks, famous restaurants, beautiful beaches, cultural sites, classic landmarks, or hiking trails. These are only a few examples of options to choose from.
- Start a group text message or email chain where you can share ideas to agree on something everyone will be interested in. Planning the road trip is a key part of deepening the bond between you and your loved ones.

- Once you've chosen your destinations, try using free road trip planners online to build an itinerary. Look up activities, must-go-to sites, and places for dining beforehand. This will save you lots of time and headaches while on your trip.
- Create a budget that calculates gas, tolls, entrance fees, meals, and lodging expenses.
- Figure out how long you want to be on the road per day, and where you will ideally be stopping for food and sleep. If you want to be proactive, book your hotels in advance to avoid the hassle. Leave room for error and flexibility in your itinerary.
- Make a packing list that's reasonable and minimalist; less is more. Assign a couple of people to make playlists to pass the time in the car.

Remember this is supposed to be a fun activity that promotes social self-care, so if you meet new friends along the way, it's okay to change up your plans a bit. Going on a road trip can get your mind off nursing and have you feeling like new when it's time to return to the bedside.

SIGN UP FOR A 5K SUPPORTING A VALUABLE CAUSE

The nursing profession expands your awareness of so many medical conditions, diseases, and world health issues. No matter your specialty, you're constantly exposed to a myriad of patient populations. This exposure may motivate you toward helping one specific population or health condition. For example, if you are a dialysis nurse, you may be a strong advocate for kidney transplant patients. One way to support your social self-care is by signing up for a 5K race that supports a cause that's close to your heart. Don't let the word *race* stop you from pursuing this mission—it's not a competition, and you can walk, run, skip, or dance to the end! But, if you're willing to train for the event, it could be that much more beneficial to your overall health. Include friends, family, and coworkers to bring everyone closer and support a meaningful cause.

You can make your training and "racing" more significant by raising awareness and fundraising for the event. You will be standing up for something you're passionate about, while promoting a healthier lifestyle. Here's how to approach the race:

- Search for a charity that supports your cause.
- If you want to fundraise, contact someone from that organization to find out how you can build a donation page online.
- Get the word out there in order to encourage others to either join you or donate money. You can bring along relatives, friends, coworkers, and community members but also make new friends along the way. Spread the word via social media.
- Create a race-day goal for yourself. If your goal is to jog the entire race without walking, there are plenty of resources online to help guide you with a training plan. If you want to raise a certain total in donations, try to reach that goal.

Anything is possible when you have the right motivation! Connecting with a cause that means a lot to you will give you built-in motivation to lend a helping hand while staying fit.

CHAPTER SIX

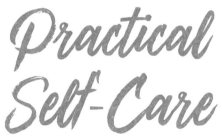

Practical Self-Care

When was the last time you felt truly in control of your life? Everything from work to school, health, and your family can feel so overwhelming. Being a nurse applies a lot of pressure on finding time to figure "life" out on your off days since you can't often squeeze in random tasks during your workdays.

So how can you regain that control? Through practical self-care, or ideas for keeping your life in order. Learning methods to organize your life can make you feel less overloaded from day to day. Activities you will find in this chapter include decluttering your house, setting a monthly savings goal, having your groceries delivered, and minimizing time wasters. You can pick and choose items that resonate with your life, or try them all! There is a strong connection between having a balanced personal life and a successful professional life, so be open-minded and get started on a more efficiently practical you.

CHECK YOUR EMAIL DURING BREAKFAST

Checking emails is usually not a lot of fun. Your inbox is probably mostly filled with spam mail, but you also get important messages mixed in that are easy to miss thanks to the sheer volume of messages. Nurses are efficient at performing multiple tasks in one sitting, and this can be one of them: Check your inbox while you have breakfast. This will allow you to go through the day's messages mindfully, but also limit the amount of time you spend doing it. Checking your inbox on a daily basis gives you the opportunity to start fresh every day. Plus, you'll be less likely to miss important messages.

As you review your messages, immediately delete unwanted emails and flag important ones as you go. If you need a lot of time to respond to a particular email, consider writing a quick response to let the person know that you saw the email and will get back to them later. Work emails tend to be filled with information, so if you need extra time to conquer these, try to do that during your actual shift! If your email system has advanced features, you might be able to personalize it to divert, say, messages about shopping or social media to one folder and messages from important senders to another folder.

MINIMIZE TIME WASTERS

It's incredible how fast time can pass you by. You can be mindlessly watching TV or scrolling through social media and before you know it, an hour has gone by. Practical self-care is about simplifying your life but also being the most efficient with the time you have. If you are not cognizant of how much time you are spending on a certain task, your day will come to an end, with only half of the things done that you had planned. Here are some fundamental tools you can use to make the most of your time any day of the week:

- First, find what your biggest time wasters are. Everyone has different vices, so it's important for you to be honest with yourself. Things like social media apps, procrastinating, games on your phone, mindlessly watching TV, and online shopping are all habits that can be minimized to regain some much-needed time.
- Cluster your tasks. (You know how you cluster care for patients? Exactly the same concept.) For example, starting a load of laundry while you wait for dinner to cook. Or checking your work email while you wait in line at the grocery store.
- Plan to get a lot accomplished when you're at your best. If you're a morning person, start laundry and dinner then. If you're a night owl, pay your bills before you go to bed.

- If you're really struggling to get things accomplished, write out a schedule for the day, hour by hour. This will hold you accountable for all of your time, while allowing you to realize how much you could get done with proper planning.
- Your phone might be a big culprit—if that's the case, try physically separating from it while you get a few things done. Social media addiction is difficult to overcome, but is vital for practical self-care. These distractions consume a lot of your time and can easily affect your mood, productivity, and self-esteem. A few helpful apps that can track your social media usage are Social Fever, Offtime, Moment, and Stay-Free. These apps also allow you to schedule "focus time," which eliminates any unwanted notifications and distractions while you work. Getting sucked into the black hole of social media can happen more often during your shift. Monitor your usage during your breaks or when you have a few minutes of downtime. You may not see how high social media usage affects your life right now, but once you minimize the time you spend scrolling, you'll notice a major difference.

You'd be surprised at the things you think you spend twenty minutes on but actually eat up hours. Recapturing even a fraction of this time can feel so rewarding!

GET RID OF CLUTTER

If the space you live in is cluttered, your mind may start to feel cluttered too. If you come home after a long shift and trip over your pet's toys, spill water on a pile of mail, and create a plastic container avalanche when cleaning up after dinner, you're only adding stress to your life.

Getting organized and controlling the clutter in your home is a key part of practical self-care. Clutter can have a significant impact on your ability to relax. You may even start avoiding certain parts of your home because of it. Getting rid of *all* clutter may seem like a daunting task, so break it down into smaller parts. Start with one room at a time, or maybe even one drawer at a time (the junk drawer is always a good place to start). It takes weeks and months for clutter to build up, so you can't expect it to all go away in one day.

Here are some tips for assessing what to do with items you're sorting through:

- Determine how often you use the item. If it's something you use once or more a week, have it in your daily living space. For things that are used a few times a year, store them somewhere more long term, like an attic, closet, or basement.
- Get rid of things that are broken, stained, ripped, outdated, or missing parts. A few examples are expired food, old receipts, dead chargers, broken jewelry, worn-out clothing, and toys with missing pieces.
- Donate items like books and clothes that are in good condition to a local charity or a friend.

Organizing and getting rid of unwanted mess is not an easy task, but it is very rewarding. You will feel a huge burden lift from your shoulders when you see a cleared-out space, and you'll likely find that you have more mental clarity for getting everything else done in your life. A clean home creates less stress in your life, which is necessary to be successful in other parts of your day.

INVEST IN A LABEL MAKER

Nurses can really appreciate consistency and organization. When you walk into a clean supply closet, where everything (for the most part) is labeled and in the correct spot, doesn't it make your whole life easier? Having things labeled really does make all the difference, so why not use this technique at home too?

A good label maker can save you so much time and energy at home. How? Here are some ideas:

- Meal prepping is ideal for a nurse's schedule. Label the containers with the date the food was prepared and the reheating instructions before you pop them into the freezer.
- Create labels to identify your cables, like chargers and USB cords, so your family members are not arguing over whose charger is missing.
- If you have a filing system for important documents, use the label maker to organize your paperwork.
- Do all the storage boxes in your attic or garage look the same? Labeling these accurately can save you a headache—and lots of time in the future when you need to find something in one of them!
- Label kids' toy storage bins so they know what goes where.

Tackle one project at a time and enjoy the satisfaction of having your home labeled!

PUT YOUR LAUNDRY AWAY

How often have you washed and dried the laundry, only for it to sit in the hamper for a few days until you grab it to wear again? Laundry is one of those tasks that can easily spiral out of control if you don't keep up with it. Between a nurse's many scrubs, compression socks, layers, and everything else, that pile of dirty clothes can get big, fast.

Instead of thinking of laundry as something you do all day on your day off, try making a different plan. Tackling one load a day can be more achievable than three or four on one day. Try getting into the habit of putting a load in the washer in the morning, transferring it to the dryer before dinner, folding it while watching TV, and putting it away shortly after. If you have a partner or children, have them help with one or two of the steps, so you don't have to take on the entire chore by yourself.

Having the laundry done and put away in the same day will have you feeling accomplished and let you go to bed with a clear mind. You won't be rummaging through the "clean hamper" for clothes the next morning!

BUY A SLOW COOKER

There's nothing better than smelling a home-cooked meal after a long day caring for patients. Unfortunately, it's not realistic that you'll always have the time to stand in front of the stove for an hour at dinnertime. A very practical solution is using a slow cooker. You can set up the cooker in the morning before you leave for work, then have a delicious meal waiting for you when you get home, hassle-free! You'll walk into mouthwatering aromas and eliminate the temptation to order out. (Take-out is usually less nutritious and more expensive, so both your body and your bank account will like this plan.)

To use a slow cooker most effectively, follow these steps:

1. Plan what you are going to make the day before. Create an ingredient list and go out and grab the items if you don't already have everything stocked at home.
2. Try to prepare ingredients the night before as well. If the meat and vegetables are already chopped, the dish will be super easy to assemble the next morning.
3. Before you leave the house, add everything to your slow cooker, cover it, and set the timer (if necessary).

This kitchen essential will also come in handy when meal prepping. You can make recipes that will yield a few meals to last you for a stretch of shifts. Slow cookers are useful for all-year-round meals too—think stews in the cool weather and burrito bowls when it's warm. Grab a cookbook filled with slow cooker options or look up a few online to get started.

PRINT OUT PHOTOS

Your phone is probably filled with great pictures you've taken over the years. But when was the last time you scrolled through them to enjoy them? Sometimes it feels great to shuffle through pictures the old-fashioned way. There's just something different about holding a photo in your hands and laughing while you share the story with a friend. This practical self-care activity will help you enjoy these photos while saving on storage space! Having the physical photos in either a box or an album can also ensure their lifespan in case your phone breaks or runs out of storage space.

There are a few ways to print photos:

- Print straight from your phone or camera to a home printer. Keep in mind that the quality might not be as good as from a store, but if getting the photos without leaving home is your priority, this option might work for you.
- Visit a store and use a kiosk to print photos. This might be a good option if you are already planning a visit to this store.
- Download an app to print photos from your phone and either pick them up at a local store or have them mailed to your home (or someone else's).

If you are in need of some positive vibes around your house, frame a few photos that bring you joy! You can even make a scrapbook or photo album to preserve all of those beautiful memories.

RUN ONE ERRAND YOU'VE BEEN PUTTING OFF

To-do lists can be helpful...but they can also get so long that you don't know where to start. Having undone errands can subconsciously make you feel unsettled and anxious, which is bad for your physical and mental well-being. On the other hand, getting things checked off that list feels so good! Especially if it's an errand you've been putting off.

Forget how long your list is, and just focus on doing one task that's been sitting on your back burner for a while now. Whether it's returning an item to the store, donating those bags of old clothes, or cleaning out your fridge, it'll be worth your time and effort to see the job completed. Sometimes thinking about what has to be done is worse than actually doing it. Schedule a time to take care of this task, and enjoy the good feelings that come with it being done!

MAKE YOUR BED

Though it may seem like a silly chore if no one's going to be in your bedroom to see it, making your bed first thing in the morning can have long-lasting benefits throughout your day. There's an immediate feeling of accomplishment, and your room just looks more put together. It's one thing that no matter what, you can control. This practical self-care activity will take just a few minutes to complete but can have a huge impact on your life.

After making your bed, you may even feel motivated to tackle another small chore. For example, with a tidy bed, you don't want to have your dirty clothes hanging off the chair, or see clutter on the nightstand. Soon enough you'll be crossing things off your to-do list left and right.

One accomplishment like this early in your morning can easily lead to a positive and productive day. Even if you've had a long and stressful day dealing with complicated patients, you can come home to a tidy bed that looks clean and inviting. That in itself will reassure you that everything will be all right, and you can get a fresh start tomorrow.

CREATE A VISION BOARD

Vision boards are a great way to manifest your goals. They're a place where you can gather visual representations of your desires so you can focus on them every day until they become reality. Visualizing the things you want to accomplish on a daily basis sends a strong message to your subconscious mind and helps you concentrate on positive things you are striving for. This activity is designed to encourage self-reflection. Here are some steps to making a vision board:

1. Start off with a brainstorming session where you picture the best life for yourself, with no limitations or restrictions. Don't limit your future; tap in to your childlike imagination and allow yourself to feel the excitement!

2. Think about broad categories, like relationships, finances, wellness, family and home, personal growth, career, travel, and hobbies. Jot down a list of goals under each category to help organize your thoughts. The more specific you are, the better results you will get.

3. Next, think about how you'd like to bring this vision board to life. You may want to get poster paper, grab some magazines and images from *Pinterest*, or create a digital board to set as your computer background. The act of physically making the vision board is also beneficial for mental and emotional self-care. It's a fun crafty project that will bring you happiness.
4. If you made a paper board, think about where you want to hang it. Make sure to choose a place that's in your daily line of sight—like in a home office or workspace, by your nightstand, or near the front door.

Visualizing your dreams can increase your motivation, confidence, and performance. Life can get so busy that it's easy to lose sight of what you're working toward and your fundamental purpose. You'll be pleasantly surprised at the joyful things you can manifest in your life just by taking the time to put them on paper.

SET A MONTHLY SAVINGS GOAL

Saving money is often easier said than done. Even if you work tons of overtime, the money can just seem to disappear if you don't plan what to do with it. Instead of automatically jumping into generating more income through overtime, take a step back and figure out exactly how much you have coming in and going out.

Many of us just go through the motions of finance without setting goals or assessing how much we spend in certain categories. For this activity, set aside time to review one month of spending and break it into categories: food, rent/mortgage, travel/commute, entertainment, and so on. Now compare what you are spending to what you are earning. What amount is realistic for you to save per month? Can you cut back on any spending areas to increase your savings instead of taking on overtime? The goal is to balance your financial goals with your physical and emotional well-being so you don't become overworked or burned out. Taking on extra hours might be a good idea to reach a short-term financial goal, like paying for a vacation or a new couch. But once you've reached that goal, be sure to give yourself a break from overtime.

If you need a hand with this goal, you can dig deeper into the topic by reading about it. A few recommended books are *The Total Money Makeover* by Dave Ramsey, *The Recovering Spender* by Lauren Greutman, *The One-Page Financial Plan* by Carl Richards, *Think and Grow Rich* by Napoleon Hill, and *Rich Dad Poor Dad* by Robert Kiyosaki.

Taking the time to truly examine your spending will make you more aware of what you can cut out and how much you can realistically be saving. You don't want to throw yourself in a state of exhaustion and risk just to make a little extra money. Figure out how you can optimize the money you are already bringing in, and come up with the best plan for yourself and your family. You will thank yourself in the future when you've saved up enough money to buy something you've been wanting!

GET ORGANIZED FOR YOUR SHIFT

A nurse's shift can be chaotic and overfilled with to-do lists. A simple way to make your work and home life easier is to get organized ahead of your shift. Having a set structure will save you lots of time and stress. There is no worse feeling than running around in chaos, and then realizing you don't have a pen or that you left your badge in your locker. Let's talk about a few ways you can coordinate yourself and your belongings ahead of time.

- Try to leave a little early for work—this will give you time for unexpected traffic and reduce the stress that comes with frantically rushing. Arriving fifteen minutes before your shift usually gives you enough time to settle yourself in.
- Once you arrive, put your things away and grab anything you might need for the day. Essentials may include pens, permanent marker, paper for reports, stethoscope, penlight, water bottle, lip balm, and ID badge.
- Glance at your patient assignment and do a quick check of orders, medications, diagnoses, and pending tests or procedures for the day. Reviewing patients' charts will prepare your mindset and help prompt certain questions you might want to ask during the handoff.

- Handoff-report time is a time when many nurses get over-whelmed, especially new nurses. Consider making your own report sheet template that will help keep your thoughts organized while getting handoff reports about your patients. Your template might include categories like patient demographics, allergies, code status, diagnoses, past medical history, past surgical history, vitals, head-to-toe assessment, lab results, IV access, drips, important medications, and plan of care. Make a report sheet that is applicable for all types of patients and that can be photocopied many times.
- Now, take a few minutes to gather your thoughts and create a functional to-do list. Multicolored pens and colorful sticky notes will help you get organized with your own color-coded system. As your shift progresses, checking things off will give you a sense of accomplishment and help guide you to what is next.
- Create alarms on your phone for any important tasks that need to be done over the course of your shift. This will prevent you from getting carried away and losing track of time.
- After your shift, clean your work area or portable computer station; get rid of any unnecessary clutter. You'll be glad you did that when you come in for your next shift.

Remaining organized before and throughout your shift will give you a sense of control and stability. A structured routine will set you up for success, while also equipping you to deal with the inevitable curveballs.

ESTABLISH A
MORNING ROUTINE

How you start your day has a huge impact on how the rest of your day will go. Snoozing the alarm clock ten times and then rushing to get out the door might be your current routine, but is it the best one? Instead of starting each new day with a negative mindset, think of it as a fresh start and a new opportunity to be extraordinary. Creating a set of habits that begin as soon as you wake up can create stability in your life that will lead to a happier and more relaxed you.

Think about what your ideal morning would look like. Would you wake up refreshed, exercise, then sit down to breakfast and coffee while reading the news? Would you meditate, then take a shower? Work backward from what you would like to achieve and create a routine that incorporates at least some of your goals while still being realistic. (Don't assume you're suddenly going to wake up chipper at 5 a.m. if you're barely able to get up at 7:45 a.m. now.)

The goal of this practical self-care activity is to be consistent for ten days straight, regardless of how you feel. You will slowly notice a shift in the direction of your days, and soon it will just become second nature. Some days you will wake up tired and unmotivated, but with a built-in morning routine, you will learn to choose discipline over emotion, and that is powerful. Soon your mornings will become more relaxed and enjoying thanks to your mindful and intentional planning!

HAVE GROCERIES DELIVERED

Some things on your to-do list need your specific attention. No one else can go to your dentist appointment, after all. But do you need to select your groceries? Maybe not. If you're strapped for time, think about getting your groceries delivered. There are many options for grocery delivery nowadays, so check out what's available in your area and try one. If you like the service you used, your items will be saved to your account, making subsequent orders even easier!

Shopping online for your food can save you time *and* money. Getting your groceries delivered gives you back the hour or two you would've spent at the store, allowing for more time meal prepping or spending time with your loved ones. You also eliminate the inevitable temptations of adding unnecessary items to your cart. If delivery services aren't available in your area, see if any stores offer curbside pickup, which is also a time-saver. If you have small children, you will also save yourself the headache of juggling between distracting them and finding everything on your list.

Once you get into a routine with your ordering, you may find this simple time-saver to be a real game changer.

USE A DRY-ERASE CALENDAR

It's challenging enough to keep up with daily to-dos, let alone the to-dos for the next few weeks. You're trying to remember scheduled shifts, bills that are due, plans with friends, birthdays, kids' activities, and appointments! Using a dry-erase calendar is a great tool for you to visualize all of these upcoming events right from a wall in your home. It will help you stay organized, aware, and productive. A dry-erase board is easy to change, update, and personalize.

Here are some tips for selecting and using a dry-erase calendar:

- Choose a board that vibes with your style and decor. Consider finding one that is magnetic so you can also post important notes, invitations, or receipts.
- Place the calendar somewhere communal, so it's in everyone's daily field of vision.

- Invest in different colored markers to help you differentiate between categories or individual family members' activities. For example, you can use red for scheduled work shifts, green for bills and paydays, blue for birthdays, black for social events, and so on.
- Cross out or erase the tasks that have been completed and days that have passed, to easily visualize your life and celebrate what you've accomplished.
- Designate a space to write overall monthly goals or plans for you and your family. This includes things like adding to your savings, making a big purchase, scheduling a nursing certification, or preparing for a big exam.

Keeping a calendar like this will help you keep track of all your events, look forward to fun plans, and reduce your stress levels significantly. So get yourself a board, hang it on your wall, and start getting organized!

WRITE OUT A WILL

No one wants to think about the end of their life. How could this possibly be a self-care activity? Well, some of us leave these important plans undone or hanging over our heads, popping up every once in a while with an "I should *really* get that done" thought. As nurses, we witness life and death on a daily basis. Because of this, we can value the importance of end-of-life care and honoring patients' wishes. Eliminate those background worries once and for all by solidifying your plans with the help of a professional.

Ask friends, colleagues, or neighbors for a recommendation of someone in your area who can help you make these plans. Here are some of the topics they can help you think about:

- Estate planning
- A last will and testament
- Healthcare proxy information
- Charitable giving or trusts

Taking the time to decide how you want to handle these sensitive topics will give you and your family peace of mind in the long run.

Index

About the Author

Xiomely Famighetti, BSN, RN, CCRN-CSC, is a critical care nurse, self-care enthusiast, and creator of the *Instagram* page @healthy.scrubs. She works with other healthcare professionals to incorporate self-care into their everyday lives. Her goal is to help other nurses create balance in their physical, emotional, and mental health. She advocates for nurses to keep their social lives flourishing, their lifestyles healthy, and their personal lives under control—all while being an extraordinary nurse.